Quality of Life
and Mental Health Care

Quality of Life and Mental Health Care

Edited by

STEFAN PRIEBE
St Bartholomew's and the Royal London School of Medicine,
University of London, UK

JOSEPH P.J. OLIVER
School of Psychiatry and Behavioural Sciences,
University of Manchester, UK

WOLFGANG KAISER
Spandau Hospital, Berlin, Germany

WRIGHTSON BIOMEDICAL PUBLISHING LTD
Petersfield, UK and Philadelphia, USA

Editorial Office:

Wrightson Biomedical Publishing Ltd
Ash Barn House, Winchester Road, Stroud,
Petersfield, Hampshire GU32 3PN, UK
Telephone: 44 (0)1730 265647
Fax: 44 (0)1730 260368

British Library Cataloguing in Publication Data
A catalogue record for this book is available from the British Library.

Library of Congress Cataloging in Publication Data
Quality of life and mental health care / edited by Stefan Priebe,
    Joseph P.J. Oliver, Wofgang Kaiser.
        p.   cm.
    Includes bibliographical references and index.
    ISBN 1-871816-40-8 (hardcover)
    1. Mental health services.   2. Quality of life.   I. Priebe,
Stefan. 1953-   ,   II. Oliver, J. P. J.'(Joseph P. J.)   III. Kaiser,
Wolfgang, 1952-   .
    [DNLM: 1. Quality of Life.   2. Mental Health Services.
3. Research.   WM 29.5 Q11 1999]
RA790.5.Q34   1999
362.2--dc21
DNLM/DLC   99-12782
For Library of Congress   CIP

ISBN 1 871816 40 8

Composition by Scribe Design, Gillingham, Kent
Printed in Great Britain by Biddles Ltd, Guildford

Contents

Contributors

A. George Awad, *Professor of Psychiatry, University of Toronto, Toronto, Ontario, Canada M5T 1R8*

Ian Daly, *Clondalkin Mental Health Services, The Village Centre, Clondalkin, Dublin 22, Eire*

Sherrill Evans, *School of Psychiatry and Behavioural Science, University of Manchester, Oxford Road, Manchester M13 9PL, UK*

Lars Hansson, *Associate Professor, Department of Clinical Neuroscience, Division of Psychiatry, University Hospital, SE-22185 Lund, Sweden*

Karin Hoffmann, *Department of Social Psychiatry, Free University of Berlin, Platanenalle 19, D-14050 Berlin, Germany*

Frank Holloway, *Consultant Psychiatrist, The Maudsley Hospital, Denmark Hill, London SE5 8AZ*

Peter Huxley, *Professor of Psychiatry, School of Psychiatry and Behavioural Science, University of Manchester, Oxford Road, Manchester M13 9PL, UK*

Wolfgang Kaiser, *Department of Adult Psychiatric Outpatients, Spandau Hospital, Griesingerstrasse 27-32, 13589 Berlin, Germany*

Susan Knight, *School of Psychiatry and Behavioural Science, University of Manchester, Oxford Road, Manchester M13 9PL, UK*

Gernot Lauer, *Bahnhofstrasse 14, D-75031 Eppingen, Germany*

Anthony F. Lehman, *Department of Psychiatry, University of Maryland at Baltimore, 685 West Baltimore Street, Baltimore, MD 21239, USA*

Joseph P.J. Oliver, *NHS Executive North West, Millenium Park, Birchwood, Warrington WA5 7QN, UK*

Stefan Priebe, *Professor of Social and Community Psychiatry, St Bartholomew's and the Royal London School of Medicine, Academic Unit, East Ham Memorial Hospital, London E7 8QR, UK*

Lakshmi N.P. Voruganti, *Assistant Professor of Psychiatry, University of Western Ontario, London, Ontario, Canada*

Richard Warner, *Mental Health Center of Boulder County, 1333 Iris Avenue, Boulder, CO 80304, USA*

Foreword

The publication of this volume marks a turning point in the literature on contemporary mental health service delivery. Its thorough examination of the many complex facets of the concept of quality of life combines with an informed, dialectical narrative to provide a timely and important treatise on a critical topic. Authors with different perspectives come together here to offer their understandings of a multidimensional concept, and, in so doing, they construct a new synthesis – a template from which more refined research and service planning can depart.

Quality of life, as a concept, has over the past two decades become a focal point for mental health services research and service planning for people who suffer from psychiatric disabilities. Some might even argue that it has assumed a position of such great importance that it affects all other areas of research and planning today. Clinical treatment plans, psychosocial rehabilitation initiatives, and efforts to enhance program relevance and consumer satisfaction are all grounded in implicit or explicit theories concerning quality of life. That quality of life is a concept with a good 'sound' – that it is in many ways a politically correct notion – in no way diminishes its usefulness. It is, in fact, at the very basis of the biopsychosocial 'model' of service delivery that dominates mental health programming today.

However, although many researchers are careful to define quality of life for their own purposes, and although there is a certain amount of face validity to a concept that appears so 'obvious', there is little standardization in its meaning. Like many other central concepts in mental health, the meaning of quality of life differs from investigator to investigator, from clinician to clinician, and, of course, from patient to patient.

All of these differences are thoroughly examined in this volume; and the contributors, instead of brandishing their own peculiar constructions of this concept, make an effort to place issues associated with ambiguity and inconsistency squarely before us. In so doing, they have produced a book that is analytical, forthright, instructive – and unique. The presentation of multiple viewpoints and the exposition of competing rationales help us to see that imprecision in the language of mental health service delivery represents more than just a failure among experts to reach agreement. In a more positive sense, it also serves the important function of permitting those with different perspectives to explore common ground.

This volume should serve as a standard for dissecting the many other concepts in mental health service delivery that are similarly important and ambiguous. Were more researchers and clinicians to shed their Humpty-Dumpty stances ('When I use a word, it means just what I choose it to mean – neither more or less!'), turf issues in service planning would be far less pervasive. Arguments could be muted, and the beginnings of consensus could emerge. And, best of all, patients could benefit from programming that minimizes simplistic approaches and increases the likelihood of achieving multidimensional and humane care.

LEONA L. BACHRACH
Consultant in Mental Health Service Planning;
formerly Research Professor of Psychiatry, Maryland

Preface

Quality of life has become an extremely fashionable and popular construct in psychiatry. While psychiatric research discovered the construct relatively late compared with psychology, sociology and other medical specialities, hundreds of studies have been published since the early 1990s and very few congresses go by without the presentation of papers which have the words 'quality of life' in the title. Improving patients' quality of life or maintaining it on as high a level as possible is now widely regarded as a central and almost the ultimate aim of mental health care, more important than conventional aims and outcome criteria such as the reduction of psychopathology or the prevention of rehospitalization. The popularity and the increasing body of research contrast with a watering-down of the term, and the potential impact of the construct for psychiatric theory and for mental health care service delivery remains somewhat unclear.

From this background, some of the researchers who have been particularly active in the field decided in 1996 to initiate an informal international research group, which was subsequently called the International Quality of Life in Mental Care Research Group. The aim of this group is to bring together different perspectives and experiences in a focused discussion and to develop further the construct and empirical research in quality of life for the benefit of mental health care.

The group consists of the authors of this book who met in Berlin in 1997 and in Dublin in 1998. It was decided to produce this book which is systematic as well as heterogeneous. It is systematic because it follows a clear outline: it starts with a chapter on the concept of quality of life, and then deals with methodological issues in its assessment. The next chapters discuss how to use quality of measures for evaluation in mental health care and for treatment and care planning. The fifth chapter is on the special subject of the relationship of quality of life and antipsychotic medication. Finally, there is a chapter on further strategies for research. The book is heterogeneous and pluralistic, providing both a main paper and a discussion paper on each subject. The authors are from six different countries and from various professional backgrounds: they are psychiatrists, psychologists and sociologists, and work as clinicians, researchers and health policy administrators. The Editors hope that the systematic approach provides an order and structure to the subject that is so often missing on conference programmes or in public discussions. The Editors also feel that the heterogeneity adequately reflects the state of the art. Even if some authors in this book may make contradictory statements, this should enable readers to attain a better understanding of the complexity of current opinions and discussions rather than a consistent, but one-sided view. The book shows that the last decade has seen substantial progress in quality of life research in psychiatry. It also demonstrates that there are many unanswered questions, most of which are not likely to have an easy answer. Those who wish to use quality of life indicators in mental health care should be fully aware of the various conceptual pitfalls and methodological shortcomings and have a realistic and adequate understanding of the limitations of its use. Only this awareness enables one to exploit the potentials of quality of life measures in mental health care. The construct remains fascinating and may be extremely beneficial to mental health services and their patients, but it must be applied with sufficient knowledge. The necessary information is available in this book.

It is hoped that students, clinicians, health administrators and managers as well as researchers who are interested in the subject will find this book a valuable basis for their own discussions and work, and a rich source of information and stimulating views.

STEFAN PRIEBE
London, Spring 1999

Acknowledgements

The Editors are extremely grateful to Marion Rex and Harshida Vadher at the Academic Unit for Social and Community Psychiatry in Newham for their invaluable support in producing this book. Their kindness and positive attitude were most encouraging, and their managerial and secretarial skills and input were essential throughout the editing process.

Abbreviations

ACT	Assertive Community Treatment
AIMS	Abnormal Involuntary Movement Scale
BDI	Beck Depression Inventory
BeBI	Berliner Bedürfnis Inventar
BELP	Berliner Lebensqualitätsprofil
BPRS	Brief Psychiatric Rating Scale
BSI	Brief Symptom Inventory
CAF	Community Adjustment Form
CAN	Camberwell Assessment of Need
DAI	Drug Attitude Inventory
GAF	Global Adaptive Functioning Scale
GHQ	General Health Questionnaire
GWBS	General Well-Being Scale
HoNOS	Health of the Nation Outcome Scale
HRQL	Health Related Quality of Life
ICM	Intensive Case Management
KLiBB	Klientenbogen zur Behandlungsbewertung
LQOLP	Lancashire Quality of Life Profile
MANSA	Manchester Short Assessment of Quality of Life
OQLQ	Oregon Quality of Life Questionnaire
PAIS	Psychosocial Adjustment to Illness Scale
POMS	Profile of Mood States
QLI	Quality of Life Interview
QLI-MH	Quality of Life Index for Mental Health
QLS	Quality of Life Self-Report
QLS-100	Quality of Life Self-Assessment
QALYs	Quality Adjusted Life Years
SAS-II	Social Adjustment Scale-II
SCL-90	Symptom Checklist
SIP-m	Modified Sickness Impact Profile
SLDS	Satisfaction with Life Domains Scale

1

Concepts of quality of life in mental health care

GERNOT LAUER

Introduction

During the last 15 years much research has been conducted under the heading 'quality of life' in psychiatry and mental health care. Surprisingly, this has often resulted in consistent empirical results (Fabian, 1990; Katschnig *et al.*, 1997; Lauer, 1993; 1994a, 1994b, 1995, 1996, 1997a, 1997b; Lauer and Schneider, 1995; Mercier and Filion, 1987). The growth of empirical knowledge has been made possible by the development of a growing number of assessments, scales and instruments within this field of research (Lauer, 1997b, 1999a; Lehman, 1996, 1997; Lehman and Burns, 1990; Priebe *et al.*, 1995; Simmons, 1994). On the other hand, there is a dearth of conceptual work and there has always been criticism concerning the lack of theory, and the shortage of clear concepts of quality of life research in psychiatry and mental health care. Renwick and Friefeld state: 'the relatively few conceptualizations of quality of life are typically not detailed or well developed. In fact, most approaches are operational in nature; that is, they are concerned with measures used to assess quality of life rather than with its conceptual foundations.' These authors conclude: 'The development of conceptual approaches to quality of life is in its infancy' (Renwick and Friefeld, 1996).

This chapter outlines some recommendations for improving the conceptual and theoretical status of quality of life research in psychiatry and mental health care. This objective is achieved in three ways. Problems concerning the definition of quality of life, related concepts, and some of the basic assumptions will be discussed. These will be followed by a review of the quality of life concepts in general literature. An overview of the approaches and concepts of quality of life in mental health care and psychiatric literature is then provided. Based on this information, some conclusions are drawn and recommendations submitted for advancing the concept of quality of life in psychiatry and mental health care.

Defining quality of life, related concepts and some basic assumptions

There is considerable agreement in the literature that there is 'no single, universally accepted definition' (Spilker, 1990) of quality of life. Different definitions lead to different concepts (Katz, 1987; Raphael, 1996) even if there is an agreement that quality of life is a multi-dimensional phenomenon and construct, aiming at a holistic or global perspective of individuals in their biopsychosocial nature (Brown et al., 1996; Fabian, 1990; Katschnig, 1997; Renwick and Brown, 1996). Often the World Health Organization's definition of health is cited as one main source for quality of life concepts: 'Health is a state of complete physical, mental and social well-being and not merely the absence of disease or infirmity' (World Health Organization, 1948). Consequently, Emerson (1985) states: 'Quality of life can be defined as the satisfaction of an individual's values, goals, and needs through the actualization of their abilities or lifestyle. Approaches to evaluating quality of life have focused upon two major sets of variables: (a) social indicators and (b) personal satisfaction, happiness, or well-being ... ' (Emerson, 1985). Pinkney et al., (1991) write: 'Quality of life has been defined as the goodness of life as measured subjectively and objectively; valid indicators of quality of life include health, physical environment, quality of housing and other material circumstances. More recently, the definition has been broadened to include living situation, use of time, community integration, financial status and safety, as well as objective measures of life satisfaction.' (Pinkney et al., 1991). Simmons reviews several definitions and states: 'In most discussions on the definition of quality of life it is acknowledged that it contains both objective and subjective elements' (Simmons, 1994). He also gives some examples of objective elements (type of housing, occupation, living arrangements, income), and states that subjective elements can only be assessed by self-reports (Simmons, 1994). Mayers (1995) undertakes a comprehensive overview for many of the approaches to definitions. The clearest, most holistic definition seen by this author, has been provided by Niemi et al.: 'Although the concept has been only loosely defined there is agreement that quality of life refers to a person's subjective well-being and life satisfaction and that it includes mental and physical health, material well-being, interpersonal relationships within and without the family, work and other activities within the community, personal development and fulfilment, and active recreation' (Niemi et al., 1988, quoted in Mayers, 1995). After discussing several theoretical approaches on the quality of life, Schipper et al. (1990), propose the following definition: 'Quality of life represents the functional effect of an illness and its consequent therapy upon a patient, as perceived by the patient. Four broad domains contribute to the overall effect: physical and occupational function; psychological state; social interaction and somatic sensation'.

When compared to related concepts, such as life satisfaction, happiness, morale, and well-being, the concept of quality of life 'appears to be a broader concept than the others from which it borrows' (Brown *et al.*, 1996). (To establish the relativity and relationship of these concepts to health, see Brickman *et al.* (1978) and Okun *et al.* (1984)).

The majority of the above cited definitions are in agreement that quality of life can be viewed at different levels (Katschnig, 1997). The first level is concerned with overall satisfaction with life. The next level covers a number of domains. Spilker (1990) distinguishes between four main domains:

1. Physical status and functional abilities,
2. Psychological status and well-being,
3. Social interactions, and
4. Economic status and factors.

Similar domains are defined by Schipper *et al.* (1990):

1. Physical and occupational function,
2. Psychological function,
3. Social interaction, and
4. Somatic sensation.

Renwick and Friefeld (1996) divide them into physical, cognitive, emotional and social domains (see other definitions cited above). The third level consists of specific single components of each domain. Domains may have different weights for different people and assessment of quality of life should be made in the first instance by the patient himself (Raphael, 1996; Simmons, 1994; Slevin *et al.*, 1988; Spilker, 1990).

Another point that receives considerable agreement in the literature is the use of qualitative approaches (Angermeyer and Kilian, 1997; Kilian, 1995; Norman and Parker, 1990; Raphael, 1996; Schneider, H.J., 1993; Simmons, 1994). Disease-specific and general non-disease-specific scales for the assessment of quality of life, should fulfil the basic psychometric requirements of reliability, validity and sensitivity (Bullinger, 1991; Fitzpatrick *et al.*, 1992; Guyatt *et al.*, 1986; Guyatt and Jaeschke, 1990; Guyatt *et al.*, 1989; Jaeschke and Guyatt, 1990; Joyce, 1988; Okun and Stock, 1987; Simmons, 1994; Slevin *et al.*, 1988).

Concepts of quality of life in the general literature

In the literature on the quality of life (Day and Jankey, 1996; Schipper *et al.*, 1990) at least 12 concepts of 'quality' are outlined. These will briefly be described and discussed in this section. The functional status and the health status approaches (Renwick and Friefeld, 1996) will not be discussed here because of their obvious limitations.

The social indicators approach

The economic approach was replaced by a social indicators approach in the 1960s (Zautra and Goodhart, 1979). Social indicators gauged the rising importance of the social welfare of a society. A major drawback of this concept is that only objectively oriented information is collected, with a focus on external factors or conditions (e.g. education, income, housing, neighbourhood, etc.). Broader population studies have been undertaken using this approach (Andrews, 1986; Andrews and Withey, 1974; Levi and Andersson, 1975). There are, however, only weak correlations between sociodemographic variables and quality of life. Furthermore, it may be criticized, 'But the selection of the domains, being researcher-driven, reflected the priorities and interests of each individual researcher, and so the indicators were far from identical and, in fact, barely resembled each other' (Day and Jankey, 1996). Najman and Levine (1981) list four principal weaknesses with the social indicators approach:

1. Vague conceptualization of the basic dimensions of what constitutes a high or low quality of life,
2. Considerable disagreement about which indicators are relevant,
3. Little concern or ability to relate inputs to outcomes, and
4. Little understanding of the association between objective conditions of life and the subjective perception of these conditions.

'In sum, studies which employ only objective indicators may have little to contribute to our understanding of the quality of life experience' (Najman and Levine, 1981). One possible solution to this problem is the use of subjective social indicators (Najman and Levine, 1981). On the other hand, information about objective social indicators is of great importance when assessing standard of living – a concept which is particularly necessary in cross-cultural studies and for mentally ill patients from lower socio-economic strata.

The psychological indicators approach

Information about quality of life from social or objective indicators is limited (Campbell *et al.*, 1976; Campbell and Rodgers, 1972). This is because they are only indirect indicators of the quality of a person's life, accounting rarely for more than 15% of the variance in quality of life. Psychological indicators depend primarily on the direct experience in a person's life, indicating how they perceive their own life (Warr, 1978). The major concepts of a subjective or psychological approach, i.e. satisfaction, happiness or well-being (Okun and Stock, 1987; Diener, 1984), account for over 50% of the variance in quality of life. 'The importance of this psychologic approach is its dual emphasis: first on patient perception, and second on the psyche as an overt contributor to physiologic outcome' (Schipper *et al.*, 1990). Cheng (1988) discusses the relevance of subjective quality of life for evaluation and programme planning. Some problems of the psychological indicators approach may be seen in the risk of social desirability, in the reporting of feelings (mood, external conditions, etc.) between persons and the loss of social indicators that reflect the real world (Day and Jankey, 1996).

An advanced example for the psychological indicators approach is given by Abbey and Andrews (1985). They propose a schematic form of causal linkages among:

1. Social psychological concepts (stress, internal control, control by others, social support, performance in personal life),
2. Psycho(patho)logical concepts (depression, anxiety), and
3. Quality of life concepts (overall quality of life, positive affect, negative affect, cognitive evaluation, self-esteem.

Objective social indicators are absent in this concept.

Personality variables

Some (psychological) approaches (Day and Jankey, 1996) include and investigate personality variables such as self-esteem, locus of control, optimism, sociability or the sense of coherence. These variables show close relationships to quality of life. In one study, perceived control and sense of coherence accounted for more than 50% of the variance in quality of life. 'If an argument could be made, that quality of life resides within the person and is not reflective of environmental conditions, programmes designed to enhance it could be curtailed', so that this approach 'could even be used as a justification for reactionary approaches to programme planning' (Day and Jankey, 1996).

The comparison approach

Some concepts (Calman, 1984; Day and Jankey, 1996; Michalos, 1986; Schipper *et al.*, 1990) postulate that there is a gap between one's present life and the standard to which one aspires. Calman (1984) proposes that quality of life measures the difference, or gap at a particular period of time between the hopes and expectations of the individual and the individual's current experiences. 'To improve the quality of life therefore, it is necessary to try to narrow the gap between hopes and aspirations, and what actually happens. The aim therefore is to try to help people to reach the goals they have set for themselves. A 'good' quality of life is therefore usually expressed in terms of satisfaction, contentment, happiness and fulfilment and the ability to cope. This definition emphasizes the importance of personal growth'

(Calman, 1984). Michalos (1986) assumes six kinds of 'gaps' in his 'multiple discrepancies' theory. Fifty-three percent of the variance is explained by the three types of comparison variables – goal-achievement gap, comparisons with previous best, and social comparisons. It can be stated that 'internal referents', such as one's comparison level and level of aspiration, are cognitive variables that mediate between objective and subjective indicators. A major problem of the comparison approach is that comparison referents are difficult to determine. 'It would seem that the number of different possibilities is endless and the probability is that many different ones come into play simultaneously' (Day and Jankey, 1996).

The medical approach

Quality of life is important apart from cure and survival. Medical decisions about different treatments may be based on quality of life differences (e.g. for hypertension: Testa *et al.*, 1993). 'Scrutiny of the medical literature finds a marked absence of quality of life theory associated with medical research' (Day and Jankey, 1996). There is an inappropriate use of spontaneously created scales, postulating the assessment of quality of life. 'Measures such as severity of pain, severity of symptoms, and exercise tolerance are accepted as measures of quality of life. The absence of a theoretical conceptualization of quality of life is lacking in virtually all studies in this area, and rarely is quality of life even defined' (Day and Jankey, 1996). Other studies include Najman and Levine (1981) and Van Dam *et al.* (1981). One further problem with this approach is the measurement of quality of life by the physician rather than by the patient (e.g. Schipper, 1983; Slevin *et al.*, 1988; Spitzer *et al.*, 1981).

The 'utility' approach

Inherent to the utility approach are 'trade-offs' between different kinds of treatments and their influence on quality of life. One important question is: What information is used by the patient in making a decision between treatments and what information is provided by the doctor to aid the patient's decision? (Schipper *et al.*, 1990).

Reintegration to normal living

Wood and Williams (1987) proposed the concept 'reintegration to normal living' as a proxy for quality of life. They included several domains in their concept: mobility, self-care abilities, daily activities, recreational activities, social activities, family roles, personal relationships, presentation of self, and general self-management skills. 'Reintegration means the ability to do what one has to do or wants to do, but it does not mean being free of disease or symptoms. Thus it is an appropriate measure for treatment outcome in chronic diseases where no cure is expected and the patient has to learn to live with the disease. The extent to which this is achieved can be thought of either in terms of reintegration, or quality of life, or both' (Schipper *et al.*, 1990).

The rehabilitation approach

In the past few years, quality of life has become an increasingly important goal of rehabilitation, and the notion of the personal nature of quality of life is now widely accepted. Quality of life is best assessed through a combination of subjective and objective measures. Quality of life is conceptualized as goodness-of-fit between a person and the environment. 'A central tenet of the model is that quality of life of a person is a function of the discrepancy between resources and stressors. Akin to gap theory, quality of life is determined by assessing the size of this discrepancy. If the discrepancy is large, quality of life is low, whereas with a small discrepancy, quality of life is high' (Day and Jankey, 1996).

This concept has several limitations. First, it is a researcher-driven approach, therefore aspects of quality of life which have some importance for the patient may be omitted. Secondly, little work has been done on definitions and conceptualization, but on the other hand there are many instruments for the assessment of quality of life. Finally, many inconsistent data have been collated from comparison studies between people with disabilities and the normal population; some of these showing no differences at all (Day and Jankey, 1996).

A community-centred concept

Following the concept of Ware (1984) (see also Schipper *et al.*, 1990), outcome variables may 'be grouped in concentric circles starting with the physiologic parameters of disease in the centre and spreading out in turn to personal functioning, psychological distress/well-being, general health perceptions, and finally social/role functioning. Ware's concept emphasizes a hierarchy by placing physical illness at the centre of the circle. Thus it opens the issue of weighting, apportioning relative values to the component parts of the quality of life construct. Also implicit in Ware's model is the effect of illness upon a community. More than a single patient's quality of life is affected by an illness. Thus, in measuring quality of life, how far can our research be extended?' (Schipper *et al.*, 1990).

A holistic model of quality of life

A qualitative research approach, the grounded-theory methodology (Glaser and Strauss, 1967), was used for the development of a holistic quality of life model. This model demonstrates the evaluation process of quality of life. It contains three core variables:

1. Personality (influenced by experiences, values, genetic disposition), influencing
2. Circumstances (influenced by domains and comparisons), leading to
3. The evaluation process (influenced by external reactions and goals and achievements), which finally leads to the quality of life (Day and Jankey, 1996).

A common problem with this approach is the conversion of qualitative data into quantitative data for comparison.

A three-element model

Felce and Perry (1995, 1996) propose a three-element model of quality of life in which personal values, life conditions, and personal satisfaction interact to determine quality of life. The personal satisfaction is assessed in a number of life domains: physical, material and social well-being, development and activity, and emotional well-being. 'Quality of life is defined as an overall general well-being that is comprised of objective and subjective evaluations of physical, material, social, and emotional well-being together with the extent of personal development and purposeful activity, all weighted by a personal set of values. Objective evaluation refers to the description of life conditions under which people live, such as health, income, housing quality, friendship network, activity, social roles, and so on. Subjective evaluation refers to personal satisfaction with such life conditions' (Felce and Perry, 1996).

This approach includes objective (social) indicators (e.g. for the conceptualization of standard of living) as well as subjective indicators of quality of life, and finds some empirical support from other studies. On the whole, it has not yet been empirically tested.

The centre for health promotion approach

Authors from the Centre for Health Promotion at the University of Toronto define quality of life as 'the degree to which the person enjoys the important possibilities of his or her life' (Renwick and Brown, 1996). The conceptual framework includes opportunities and constraints that may occur in a person's life by chance or by choice. The person is seen as living in an environmental context. The different parts of quality of life are seen in three components and their subcomponents:

1. Being (the person as an individual – physical, psychological, spiritual);

2. Belonging (how environments and others fit with person – physical, social, community);
3. Becoming (what person does to achieve hopes, goals, aspirations – practical, leisure, growth (Renwick and Brown, 1996).

Renwick and Brown (1996) have reported some of the empirical studies based on this approach and agree that further research is required.

Concepts of quality of life in psychiatry and mental health care

Over the past few years, quality of life has become an important goal for psychiatric rehabilitation (Priebe, 1994; Sartorius, 1992). One of the aims of psychiatric rehabilitation is: 'To improve the person's overall sense of well-being' (Bridges *et al.*, 1994; Lauer, 1997c). About 15 years ago, Schulberg and Bromet (1981) recommended: 'When valid and reliable instruments are available for assessing a patient's quality of life, i.e. a composite of the preceding variables, such analyses should be included in this first priority category'. A decade later other authors complained that: 'Early attempts to define and measure quality of life in the chronically mentally ill were clinically useful ... , but either did not have a comprehensive model of quality of life or did not report psychometric properties of the instruments' (Levitt *et al.*, 1990).

Today, a large number of instruments for the assessment of quality of life in psychiatry are being developed (Lauer, 1997b, 1999; Lehman, 1996, 1997; Lehman and Burns, 1990; Simmons, 1994), but nevertheless the field shows theoretical weaknesses. Several researchers have commented on the concept of quality of life in psychiatry and mental health care, but the growth of such concepts is only marginally based on the development of quality of life in the general literature (see above). In this section, five concepts of the quality of life have been developed mainly in psychiatry and mental health care. These will be critically reviewed. Finally, a special issue, medications and quality of life will be discussed.

The social indicators approach

There are some relationships between social indicators (e.g. unemployment; Brenner, 1973) and mental health (e.g. admissions, services utilization, hospitalization rates). In an earlier paper on the measurement of rehabilitation outcome in schizophrenia (under the heading 'patient quality of life'), only objective and social indicators are listed: number of hours per week spent alone, number of social contacts per week, number of club or organizational meetings attended, number of recreational/sports activities per month, number of conversations per week, number of new items of clothing per year, and number of hot meals eaten per week (Anthony *et al.*, 1978). One major problem with this approach is the lack of specificity and a highly uncertain validity. 'Many indicators are used as surrogates of psychological well-being, however, even though they lack a basic anchor in the human meaning of social events' (Zautra and Goodhart, 1979). On the other hand, some demographic variables are correlated with psychological indicators of quality of life, i.e. socioeconomic status, age, marital status or sex.

An example of the social indicators approach in psychiatry is given Fabian's (1989) investigatory work, on gender and race and their impact on subjective quality of life – as assessed by the Quality of Life Interview (QLI; Lehman, 1988) – of psychiatric patients.

The psychological indicators approach

Important for the psychological indicators approach are the subjective reactions to life experiences. Shadish *et al.* (1985) compared different methods in the assessment of quality of life in different groups of patients. Cheng (1988) discusses the relevance of subjective quality of life for the evaluation and programme planning of community support programmes for chronic mental patients. Corrigan and Buican (1995) investigated the construct validity of subjective quality of life. 'Findings from a multiple regression analysis suggested that depression, social adjustment, size of the support network, and verbal intelligence are independently associated with quality of life. This suggests that quality of life is not redundant with the anhedonia common to depression' (Corrigan and Buican, 1995).

Several models can be subsumed to the psychological indicators approach. The Gothenburg group (Malm *et al.*, 1981) discussed the schizophrenic needs approach. This is when the schizophrenic patient is regarded as a complete human being and is involved in four overlapping systems, being the health care, rehabilitation, family and community humanitary systems (May, 1986). These authors' quality of life concept is merely based on the needs of the recovering patient with schizophrenia: medical care, human relationships, material quality of life, communication and transport services, work and work conditions, safety, knowledge, education, leisure and recreation, and inner experience.

A life-crisis model is based on Caplan's (1994) conceptual model of primary prevention. The basic thought is that a crisis can either promote or hinder adjustment, depending upon how the crisis is resolved. Social support and supply may help to resolve the problems. Handal and Moore (1987) tested Caplan's supply model with a group of $N=108$ non-psychiatric probands. For each of three supply scales the group with the lowest access to physical, psychosocial, and sociocultural supplies reported significantly less life satisfaction and significantly more psychological distress than the high access group.

Competency models view people as active agents who govern their own lives. The core variables of competency models may be personal autonomy (Hachey and Mercier, 1993; Mercier and King, 1994) or self-esteem and self-efficacy (Arns and Linney, 1993; Barry, 1997).

Hachey and Mercier (1993) propose a model with three sets of variables influencing quality of life:

1. Individual characteristics,
2. Living conditions, and
3. Utilization of services.

Based on this model, a later study using pathanalytic methods, showed that 'results indicate that greater autonomy is significantly associated with greater perceived quality of life and that greater quality of life ratings are associated with greater community tenure' (Mercier and King, 1994). Self-esteem and self-efficacy are the core variables of a model proposed by Arns and Linney (1993). They propose a rehabilitation outcome model containing several factors:

1. Individual factors and the psychosocial rehabilitation process; which influences
2. Community tenure, change in residential status, and a change in vocational status. The latter two variables are hypothesized to influence
3. Self-esteem and self-efficacy. These two variables are largely influencing
4. Life satisfaction (Arns and Linney, 1993). In their empirical investigation it is demonstrated 'that changes in vocational status have a significant impact on the self-concepts and life satisfaction of persons with severe and persistent mental disabilities' (Arns and Linney, 1993). In another study, Lauer and Sellmann (1993) found strong correlations between self-esteem and quality of life in people with schizophrenia, and concluded that just as in the normal population, self-esteem is a strong predictor of quality of life in chronically mentally ill patients.

A positive mental health model includes two independent sets of needs: avoidance of or adjustment to painful life experiences, and developing and sustaining life satisfaction by increasing competence, skills, and mastery over the environment (for details see Zautra and Goodhart, 1979).

All models of the psychological indicators approach share some limitations: social desirability response bias, idiosyncrasy in reports of feeling states, and the question of the adequacy of psychological indicators. On the other hand, there may be useful applications of the psychological indicators approach. For example, quality of life data derived from psychological indicators may help confirm social indicator reports of service needs among community groups and neighbourhoods.

Adaptive functioning models

In addition to the social and psychological indicator approaches, Schalock *et al.* (1989) mention goodness-of-fit or social policy models. These approaches often are referred to under the heading of adaptive functioning models (Fabian, 1990). 'They point out that two important variables in mental health assessment are individual satisfaction and individual performance in relation to social expectations. Life and the environment present opportunities through which the person may satisfy needs, both materially and socially, but which also present demands and responsibilities. The extent to which a person enjoys a reasonable or high quality of life will depend on the degree to which he or she can meet the demands of life, and hence achieve fulfilment of need and satisfaction' (Simmons, 1994). At least three adaptive functioning models in psychiatry and mental health care are to be considered. The model of Baker and Intagliata (1982) distinguishes four foci:

Focus I: environmental system (social indicators),
Focus II: experienced environment (psychological indicators – 14 domains),
Focus III: bio-psycho system (health, well-being, and needs), and
Focus IV: behaviour (self-management and adaptation).

Focus II and Focus III are within the person, and comparisons (against standards, levels of adaptation) are made between both these foci. This model is partially tested and supported by findings of a positive relationship between social support and perceived quality of life (Baker *et al.*, 1992).

Psychiatric thoughts, the social adaptation perspective, role theory, and results of empirical studies on quality of life are combined in the model of Bigelow *et al.* (1982) (see also Angermeyer and Kilian, 1997). Their concept includes social indicators (opportunity structure), and psychological variables (happiness, satisfaction). They also conceptualize opportunities and demands of the environment, and abilities, performance and satisfaction of the individual. 'The client's needs are reflected in this system under the heading of satisfaction, and society's needs are under the heading of performance. Together, they constitute adjustment' (Bigelow *et al.*, 1982). In their later paper (Bigelow *et al.*, 1991) it is stated: 'Our concept of quality of life is drawn largely from need (Maslow, 1954) and role theories. Quality of life, as researchers view it, comes out of a social contract-fulfilment of needs in exchange for meeting of demands which society places upon its members. Needs are fulfilled through opportunities presented by the social environment. Demands are met through the exercise of basic psychological abilities – cognition, affect, perception, and motor' (Bigelow *et al.*, 1991).

A further example of adaptive functioning models is probably illustrated in the three-dimensional model (Franklin *et al.*, 1986). Besides objective social indicators in different domains and the subjective assessment of those domains (two-part model, or two-domain model: Gannon *et al.*, 1992), adaptation to life situations is assessed. The following assumptions for the three-dimensional model are made:

1. Life situations (objective indicators): housing (type), living arrangements (with whom), social relations (number of friends), leisure (number of activities), income (individual monthly income), employment (employed/unemployed);
2. Subjective assessment of life situations: satisfaction with housing, living arrangements, social relations, leisure, income, employment;
3. Adaptation to living situations: activities of daily living, affect balance, self-esteem;
4. Other factors (unspecified; for details see Franklin *et al.*, 1986).

This approach was empirically tested by comparing an experimental case management group with a control group, both showing only marginal differences after 12 months (Franklin *et al.*, 1987).

One socio-ecological model of coping (Kearns *et al.*, 1987) proposes a conceptual framework containing eight sets of variables:

1. Personal characteristics (employment, gender, income, age),
2. Psychiatric profile (diagnosis),
3. Psychiatric services (programme participation),
4. Housing situation (location, cost, type),
5. Social support network (formal aftercare, informal support),
6. Lifestyle (activities, use of time),
7. Beliefs, and
8. Client outcomes (coping, satisfaction, community tenure) (Kearns *et al.*, 1987).

In a Canadian study (Caron *et al.*, 1998), the variable of social support is included in the conceptual framework of quality of life.

In a later publication by the Gothenburg group (Skantze and Malm, 1994) a gap theory is shown. 'According to a vulnerability–stress–coping–quality of life model, quality of life and well-being are influenced by the dynamic gap between personal aspirations, dreams, and hopes on the one hand, and perceived reality on the other. Since individual preferences and aspirations, dreams, and ambitions differ considerably depending on genetic factors, life experiences, and perceptions of reality, a person's quality of life can be judged only subjectively' (Skantze and Malm, 1994).

Combined approaches: social and psychological indicators

In psychiatry and mental health care, certain concepts include objective social indicators as well as subjective psychological indicators of quality of life. In two studies from the Gothenburg group (Skantze *et al.*, 1990; Skantze *et al.*, 1992) four sets of variables are taken into account:

1. Personal characteristics,
2. Standard of living – objective,
3. Quality of life – subjective, and
4. Welfare.

'There was no significant association between patients' overall perception of their quality of life and their total standard of living ($r=0.19$, $p>0.10$) despite the large variance found in the QLS' (Quality of Life Self-Report, Skantze *et al.*, 1992).

   Perhaps the most prominent combined approach comes from Lehman (1983a) whose concept is based on general population studies (Andrews and Withey, 1976; Campbell *et al.*, 1976). It makes the central points that (i) ultimately, quality of life is a subjective matter, reflected in a sense of global well-being, and (ii) this experience depends on at least three types of variables: (a) personal characteristics, such as age and sex, (b) objective quality of life in various domains of life, such as income level, and (c) subjective quality of life in these same life domains, such as satisfaction with income. This quality of life model contrasts with the approach more commonly used for assessing quality of life in which only objective life conditions are measured; subjective quality of life is then inferred from these observations. Unfortunately, the literature indicates that objective quality of life indicators bear at best modest relationship to life satisfaction in the general population and that subjective quality of life indicators are needed to obtain a more comprehensive assessment of quality of life. It has been suggested that these shortcomings of objective quality of life indicators may be even more marked among persons leading atypical life-styles, such as chronic mentally ill patients (Lehman, 1983a). Eight domains are included in this model: living situation, family, social relations, leisure, work, law-safety, finances, and health. The predicted variance by the three types of variables is:

1. Personal characteristics: 4–7%; in addition to
2. Objective quality of life indicators: 14–23%, and
3. Subjective quality of life indicators: 48–58% (Lehman, 1983a).

This approach and the Quality of Life Interview (QLI; Lehman, 1988) stimulated many empirical studies (Aberg-Wistedt *et al.*, 1995; Barry and Crosby, 1996; Barry *et al.*, 1993; Champney and Dzurec, 1992; Huxley and Warner, 1992; Kaiser *et al.*, 1996; Lehman *et al.*, 1986, 1991, 1992; Levitt *et al.*, 1990; Okin and Pearsall, 1993; Oliver and Mohamad, 1992; Simpson *et al.*, 1989; Vandiver *et al.*, 1993; Warner and Huxley, 1993). Problems of this approach may arise when patients from different settings, facilities and programmes are compared. One example of the different meaning of objective and subjective indicators using this model and parts of the Quality of Life Interview (Lehman, 1988), is given by the study of Sullivan *et al.* (1991). 'Thus if the Mississippian's relatively high quality of life ratings were related to their living with family members, it is unlikely that the ratings were due to better living circumstances. The relatively high ratings are more likely attributable to factors such as emotional or instrumental social support' (Sullivan *et al.*, 1991). Another point is the relationship of psychiatric diagnoses and psychopathology – both explicitly not included in the model – to quality of life (Lehman, 1983b; Simpson *et al.*, 1989; Warner and Huxley, 1993).

Other approaches

Several other approaches have been proposed in the field of psychiatry and mental health care, sometimes focusing on different aspects of quality of life (Katschnig *et al.*, 1997). Some of them will be briefly presented below.

Earls and Nelson (1988) tested some hypotheses derived from the motivation–hygiene theory. They demonstrated that housing and social support would be differently related to the psychological well-being assessed in terms of the positive and negative affect on long-term psychiatric patients.

Contrary to the concept of family burden, the psychological well-being of family members and relatives of schizophrenics is focused on in the study by Oldridge and Hughes (1992). Simon (1997) summarizes the results on studies concerning the quality of life of relatives of mentally ill persons.

The topic of quality of life and cost-effectiveness is dealt with in several papers (Meltzer *et al.*, 1993; Salvador-Carulla, 1997; Wilkinson *et al.*, 1992; Williams *et al.*, 1992). Coid (1993) discusses philosophical and legal problems of the quality of life of detained psychiatric patients.

Corten *et al.* (1994) present a factor analytical model, containing three factors:

1. Hedonistic factor,
2. Achievement factor, and
3. Confirmity factor.

From their database, they conclude that: 'Contrary to the hypothesis of the Social Indicators movement, it appeared that items related to the objective satisfaction of needs were not related to items of the subjective quality of life' (Corten *et al.*, 1994).

Schneider (1993), from the point of view of hermeneutic philosophy, criticizes empirical quality of life research. Likewise Kilian (1995) and Angermeyer and Kilian (1997) shed critical light on the one-sided quantitative methodological orientation of quality of life research in psychiatry. They propose a dynamic model of subjective quality of life, combining both qualitative and quantitative research methods (Angermeyer and Kilian, 1997;

Kilian, 1995). Recently another qualitative approach to the quality of life of people with schizophrenia has been proposed (Kühn *et al.*, 1997).

Special issue: medications and quality of life

In an early paper, Diamond (1985) discusses that subjective neuroleptic side-effects – not only objectively observed ones (dystonia, akathisia, tardive dyskinesia, etc., for reviews see Casey, 1994; King, 1990; Sullivan and Lukoff, 1990) – may influence the patient's quality of life and lead to non-compliance (Corrigan *et al.*, 1990). 'We must learn to balance discrepancies between the clinician's and the patient's view of cost and benefit, their evaluation of unreasonable risk, and their view of treatment goals. Researchers must listen to our patients before they will listen to us' (Diamond, 1985). In chronic somatic disorders, the impact of side-effects of medications on quality of life is important for treatment decisions (e.g. Croog *et al.*, 1986; Peduzzi *et al.*, 1987; Testa *et al.*, 1993). On the other hand, Lepkifker *et al.*, (1988) found no interference by lithium on the life satisfaction in affective patients. For patients with schizophrenia, Awad (1992) proposes a model containing three major determinants: (i) symptoms, (ii) side-effects, (iii) psychosocial performance, and as a fourth factor, the subjective interpretation of the medicated state may be added. Another methodological solution and model is provided by Bagne and Lewis (1992). Awad and Hogan (1994) state: 'it is surprising that not much attention has been given to systematic evaluation of the quality of life of schizophrenic patients on neuroleptics nor in clinical trials of new neuroleptics', and note a 'lack of a conceptual model for quality of life on neuroleptics' (Awad and Hogan, 1994). Angermeyer (1994) proposes a model based on the theory of reasoned action (Ajzen and Fishbein, 1980) for the explanation of subjectively impaired quality of life by neuroleptics. This model also allows a better understanding of non-compliance in patients with schizophrenia. Angermeyer and Katschnig (1997) discuss some side-effects of different classes of psychotropic drugs which may have implications for quality of life.

Several studies found negative correlations between side-effects and quality of life (Lauer and Bähr, 1988: $r=-0.50$, $p<0.01$; Lauer and Stegmüller-Koenemund, 1994: $r=-0.51$, $p<0.01$ for social contact, $r=-0.44$, $p<0.01$ for health, $r=-0.43$, $p<0.01$ for safety, $r=-0.39$, $p<0.05$ for living situation, $r=-0.38$, $p<0.05$ for work and employment; Sullivan *et al.*, 1992: $r=-0.28$, $p<0.05$). In an Austrian study (Hinterhuber *et al.*, 1995), it was found that side-effects of neuroleptics diminished the quality of life of people with schizophrenia by about 15%. Franz *et al.* (1996) reported a better quality of life in three of the four scales of the Munchner Lebensqualitts Dimensionenliste for a group of patients on atypical neuroleptics (clozapine, zotepin, risperdone). In a recent study (Lauer, 1997d) comparing two groups of $N=30$ schizophrenics on classic neuroleptics or on clozapine, the group treated with clozapine expressed a better quality of life in four of nine domains: social contacts, leisure, safety and health. Thus, concepts of quality of life in psychiatry and mental health care should include the topic of medication and its impact on the individual's quality of life.

Conclusions and recommendations

Many psychiatric and non-psychiatric authors complain of a lack in the development of concepts in quality of life research. Several conclusions and recommendations from earlier sections of this chapter can be made.

1. It is good to have 'no single, universally accepted definition' (Spilker, 1990) of quality of life. This helps us to keep the construct of quality of life open – as is undertaken with other psychological constructs, for example, intelligence. On the other hand, different definitions lead to different concepts.
2. There is agreement that quality of life contains important subjective concepts, e.g. satisfaction, and there is also agreement that objective variables, e.g. standard of living, are necessary.
3. A domain-structure with different domains from different authors and in different instruments is helpful. The concrete number, headings, and content of the domains may be discussed.
4. Quality of life has a hierarchical structure, including other concepts, such as well-being, satisfaction with life, etc.
5. Qualitative approaches, e.g. using in-depth interviews and content-analytic methods, are helpful for some minor and underdeveloped fields of interest. One possible example is the side-effects of medications on quality of life.
6. General quality of life literature and research offers limitations and chances for psychiatry and mental health care. The chances may be seen in the cited social-psychological and psychological concepts (e.g. Abbey and Andrews, 1985). Also some personality variables, used in general quality of life concepts, e.g. self-esteem, are helpful and fruitful in psychiatry (Arns and Linney, 1993; Lauer and Sellmann, 1993).
7. The comparison approach should be further developed in psychiatry and mental health care. On the other hand, bearing in mind the ambivalence of some patients with schizophrenia, it may be too difficult to assess too complicated internal referents.
8. From the medical approach researchers can learn to avoid some mistakes and serious conceptual problems.
9. Ideas from the reintegration to normal living approach, the rehabilitation approach and Ware's (1984) community centred concept may help

us to overlook the boundaries of our social-psychiatric positions. At this point, it is necessary to discuss the question of disease-specific or generic quality of life assessments.

10. The relationship of quality of life to other subjective concepts, i.e. satisfaction with treatment, satisfaction with care providers, etc.

11. If researchers decide to use adaptive functioning models, especially gap theories, then they should integrate the great body of theory and empirical results from social psychology (e.g. theory of social comparison, adaptation-level theory, etc.).

12. Caplan's (1994) model may help us to close the gaps between psychiatric patients in the community and the normal population. This also focuses on the construct of social support as an important variable to be included in quality of life concepts (see also Caron et al., 1998; Kearns et al., 1987).

13. The three-dimensional model (Franklin et al., 1986) once again emphasizes the relevance of subjective constructs such as self-esteem (see also Arns and Linney, 1993, Lauer and Sellmann, 1993).

14. Service participation and the impact of different programmes on different patients are to be studied longitudinally (e.g. Mechanic, 1997; Mercier and King, 1994).

15. Complex models (e.g. Baker and Intagliata, 1982) need complex assessments and methods. Pragmatic research may be more fruitful.

16. Combined approaches, using social and psychological indicators (e.g. Barry, 1997; Lehman, 1983a) are helpful, especially for cross-cultural comparisons. Social indicators are of great relevance to cross-cultural quality of life studies (e.g. Bullinger et al., 1993; Vandiver et al., 1993; Warner and Huxley, 1993).

17. Conceptual thoughts and empirical results are required on the relationship of different psychopathologies (depression, anxiety, compulsion, positive symptoms, negative symptoms) to quality of life (Katschnig, 1997). One hypothesis may be that depression and anxiety will affect quality of life more than the positive and negative symptoms of schizophrenia which may have little or no effect (e.g. Lauer, 1994b).

18. The same is true for the problem of quality of life and side-effects of different medications (low and high potent typical neuroleptics, atypical neuroleptics, tricyclic antidepressants, selective serotonin reuptake inhibitors, benzodiazepines, etc.; see also Angermeyer and Katschnig, 1997). First results suggest that patients with schizophrenia treated with atypical neuroleptics experience a better quality of life (e.g. Lauer, 1997d).

19. Quality of life should be related to other outcome variables (e.g. Avison and Speechley, 1987: readmission to the hospital, community tenure, core role performance, social adjustment, current level of symptoms, global outcome).

1: Discussion

Advancing the concepts of quality of life

LARS HANSSON

Introduction

The thorough review of different traditions in the development of the quality of life concept presented in the preceding chapter by Gernot Lauer shows that so far there has not been an advancement of the concept of quality of life, but rather an accumulation of a number of separate but not consistent concepts and definitions. A number of questions and problems arise from the review, which may be of importance in a discussion on the advancement of the quality of life concept within the field of mental health care.

In this chapter, the following topics will be discussed: (i) the state of the art of the concept of quality of life, (ii) the need for a consensus on the concept, (iii) the need for a theoretical framework of quality of life, (iv) the relationship between subjective and objective quality of life, (v) the relationship between psychopathology and subjective quality of life, and (vi) the relationship between quality of life and other outcome measures.

The state of the art of the concept

Lauer's review shows with great clarity that quality of life during the last three decades has been defined in many ways and within various theoretical frameworks. In a way this is not astonishing because, as far as health care research is concerned, this is well in line with other areas of measures or constructs, where a diversity of instruments is used, and where differences in the underlying conceptualization exist. Although from a researcher's point of view, this raises methodological problems, problems of choice, and difficulties in comparing results from studies, it is not necessarily a general problem. One obvious reason for the diversity of quality of life concepts and definitions is that they have been developed in different contexts and with differences in objectives, research methodology and focus of investigation. A general classification or taxonomy of quality of life definitions would consist of five broad categories, of which four are based on expert, *a priori* or professional definitions (Farquahar, 1995). There are global definitions, component definitions, combinations of these two, and focused definitions. A fifth category including empirically derived, individualized, or lay definitions also exists.

Global definitions seem historically to be quite common. However, because of their generality they tell us little about possible components of quality of life or how researchers should operationalize the concept. These general definitions often include assumptions concerning well-being, satisfaction or dissatisfaction and/or happiness or unhappiness with life.

Component definitions break down the quality of life concept into components or domains, or identify a number of characteristics essential in the evaluation of quality of life. This category of definitions takes us a step further towards an operationalization of the concept. Sometimes these definitions merely list domains of interest without any reference to a specific theory, or without any explicit ideas concerning the interrelationship between these life domains. These definitions might be further divided into general definitions or definitions specific to a certain research area or research topic, such as the quality of life of the elderly or the mentally ill. A third category consists of combinations of the two above categories; the definitions contain a global part but also include a number of derived components.

Focused definitions refer only to one or a small number of components of quality of life. These might be divided into explicit focused definitions such as in the case of 'health related quality of life', and implicit focused definitions where it is not made clear that the definition is not comprehensive, and that only a few components of a more global concept are included.

All these four types of definition are developed from a professional/expert perspective and may at times have a hypothetical or theoretical origin. However, a central issue in defining quality of life lies in the choice of perspective. A fifth category of definitions which might be labelled lay definitions, is based on empirical investigations in defined populations, of what constitutes the components of quality of life. Definitions evolving from this approach have been proposed to ensure a greater appropriateness and acceptability, and to a higher degree reflect the individual's priorities and preferences.

The review by Lauer gives the impression that it is still true that there are almost as many quality of life definitions as there are quality of life researchers. However, it seems that there is an emerging consensus, if not on a conceptual level, about the general dimensions of quality of life and its determinants. There has been a general trend from more objectively defined concepts, including the social indicators movement, towards the understanding of quality of life as largely determined by the individual's subjective experiences of life and life conditions. Therefore it is nowadays mostly pointed out that personal characteristics, role functioning, objective social and other life conditions, together with the subjective experience of different life domains would form a comprehensive determinant or indicator of an individual's quality of life. The relative importance of these factors is perhaps not yet settled, but it is stressed that subjective experiences or life satisfaction play a major role (Oliver *et al.*, 1997).

The need for a consensus

There is no consensus on the quality of life concept and Lauer concludes that this is a good thing. A circumstance partly explaining the current diversity of quality of life concepts and measures, is the multidisciplinary nature of the field. This field has stimulated economists, psychologists, philosophers, sociologists, political scientists, health care researchers and many others. It is therefore not astonishing that this has led to a variation in the aspects or domains of quality of life that specific research groups have emphasized. This variation reflects differences in theory building and focus of research. Cultural and subcultural differences may also be of importance. An example of the latter is that, looking at the history of quality of life research, American researchers have, more than European researchers, stressed subjectivity and life satisfaction as important features of quality of life. The Scandinavian research tradition has generally relied more on objectively defined indicators, which sometimes may be defined more adequately as welfare research, and there are other European research groups which have focused more on a needs approach.

Nevertheless, there has been a concern about the lack of consensus regarding the concept. When this discussion has touched upon the vagueness and ambiguity of the concept it has been a good thing, since an increased clarity of the concept is warranted. Due to the varying interests in and purposes of the development of quality of life measures, it may be that the search for a golden standard of an overall quality of life concept is a search in vain. It may not even be desirable, because considering the many stakeholders in the field, the result of such a development would be a definition which is opposed by very few but, on the other hand, necessarily so general and superficial that it would not be instrumentally very useful. Probably it would be more fruitful to engage in a matching procedure, where further development of the concept and measures should be based on a more thorough match between the quality of life concept used, the aims and focus of the research, the population studied, the purpose of specific investigations, and the users of empirical findings. This would also be an approach which is well in line with current approaches when it comes to general health care research methodology. Of course this raises the question about whether generic concepts and measures are preferable to population-specific, disease-specific or otherwise focused approaches.

The need for a theoretical framework

Given the rather confusing discussion on how quality of life should be defined, and the variety of theories used in developing concepts and measures, one might give some consideration to the need to advance the theoretical framework of quality of life. It seems that, so far, there have, on the one hand, been groups which have been engaged in discussions of the concept and its content. On the other hand, there has been an empirical tradition of investigating quality of life, often ignoring any more elaborate concerns about theories and concepts of quality of life. This also goes for investigations of quality of life of the mentally ill, as noted by Barry and Zissi (1997) in a recent review. A critical appraisal of the quality of quality of life research in health care performed by Gill and Feinstein (1994), revealed that out of 75 studies using quality of life measures, where the included studies were randomly chosen from a database search, quality of life was conceptually defined in only 15% of the studies. Reasons for selecting the chosen quality of life instrument were given in 36% of the studies and the targeted domains of quality of life were identified in 47% of the studies. If these results are representative, it seems that empirical studies of quality of life are, to a large extent, conducted without any conceptual or theoretical preferences. If this is the case, which aspects are good or bad? Of course, a theory-based approach may help to analyse and interpret results from studies. Empirical findings may also be used to verify or reject hypotheses derived from theory, and thereby be of help in a further advancement of the concept.

However, there is a more fundamental discussion in connection with this that would be of more interest. Regardless of perspective, quality of life is a value-loaded concept in terms of its definition and operationalization. Any theory based, or *a priori*, definition is at least implicitly relying on some values and beliefs of what constitutes the essential qualities of life, and the dimensions along which they should be assessed. It would perhaps be fruitful for the advancement of this field to embark on a discussion of the origins and appropriateness of these basic values and beliefs. Initially, what might be included in such a discussion are the values of the researcher. On what grounds are certain domains of life included and chosen for measurement? This discussion becomes important also in light of the fact that domains and items often are chosen not for their specific psychometric properties but rather due to what has been labelled clinimetrics. A question secondary to this concerns the weighting of different domains or items in a quality of life measure. Should different items in a measure have the same influence, or should they be differently weighted in order to reflect differences in perceived importance or priorities of the individual? These matters could of course be discussed within a statistical framework, but there is also an obvious and important value-based and conceptual dimension to it.

Secondly, the values and preferences of the individual should be considered in this discussion. As an example, is it beneficial for all people to have many social relations, or is it bad for some? Are social relations equally important to all people, or are they very important for some individuals and of minor importance for others? A person who values highly a top income needs a top income to be satisfied with his quality of life. On the other hand, the individual who does not care much about money could have all the money in the world and still perceive a low quality of life. The question arising from these examples concerns how the values, preferences and priorities of the individual regarding quality of life may be integrated in a quality of life concept and its definition.

A discussion of this also touches upon whether quality of life should be considered a trait or a state, not with regard to its sensitivity to changes in life, but whether it is based on an enduring and stable set of the individual's values. Does the individual's evaluation of what is considered important in life change with changes in life conditions due to adaptation processes, changes in aspirations and expectations, or is it stable? Deinstitutionalized patients have for example been shown to experience an increased satisfaction with life, but are these findings stable over time, or would long-term follow-ups show a different pattern? How this is viewed may affect the conclusions drawn from such studies.

An interesting approach in building a theoretical model has been proposed by Barry (1997). This mediational model of quality of life is an effort to link self-related constructs such as self-esteem and self-efficacy to the subjective evaluation of quality of life. It also proposes that certain expectations, aspirations and comparison standards mediate the evaluation of objective life conditions. An empirical study performed to test the model gave a support for the link between self-esteem and subjective quality of life, while no relationship between objective quality of life indicators and subjective quality of life was found (Zissi et al.,1998).

Subjective and objective quality of life

A central issue in quality of life research has been: who is to define what quality of life is and what its components are, and who should assess it? There has been an increased awareness that objective indicators may tell us little about a person's quality of life. There is subjectivity to the concept, which has led to the conclusion that an individual's subjective and inner experiences of the life situation in different domains are a central feature of the quality of life. But there are some findings that may require a further discussion on the nature of subjective quality of life and its relationship to objective life conditions. How should researchers understand a lack of association between objective indicators of quality of life and subjective quality of life? How should researchers interpret an association of poor objective life conditions with a high satisfaction with life? Why is it that changes in objective life conditions may not be reflected in changes in life satisfaction, or that intervention studies do not show changes in subjective quality of life? Does this throw a shadow on the validity of the concept of subjective quality of life, or are researchers using measures not sensitive to changes in objective life conditions? It has also been proposed that life satisfaction in different domains does not have any clear-cut objective counterparts. There are many ways to interpret findings like these and one comment, which may be of importance, concerns the way subjective quality of life is generally defined and measured. Subjective quality of life is generally defined as the individual's satisfaction with a number of *a priori* set life domains, compiled from an expert, normative or hypothetical perspective. This means that, although the individual is performing assessments of his subjective satisfaction with life, he has no influence on what domains to evaluate, nor may the individual express the relative preferences concerning the importance of these domains, or items tapping satisfaction in these domains. This is a rather paternalistic way of evaluating subjective quality of life, reflecting different kinds of societal norms, which affects the content validity of the construct. There would be gains to be made from mainly qualitative research investigating what domains should be included, and the relative importance of them. Furthermore, in order to reflect individual priorities, investigations where individual determinants of subjective quality of life are used, instead of or in addition to standard domains, might also be useful (Calman, 1984; Barry and Zissi, 1997).

The relationship between psychopathology and subjective quality of life

Most studies investigating this relationship have found an association between psychopathology in terms of psychiatric symptoms, and the subjective quality of life. This association has especially been pointed out regarding depressed mood and anxiety (Corrigan and Buican, 1995; Lehman, 1988; Sullivan *et al.*, 1992). Results concerning the relationship between quality of life and psychotic symptoms have been more mixed. It also seems that self-report measures of symptoms are more related to subjective quality of life than objective interview-based measures of psychopathology. What conclusions can be drawn from findings that depressed patients show lower levels of subjective quality of life than other groups of psychiatric patients? Is it illness-related insofar as the perception of life is distorted, which makes satisfaction with life lower than it, in some sense, really is, or should researchers take these perceptions at face value and accept them as the inner experiences of different life domains? This is not to say that there are not situations where a severe psychopathology may prohibit an individual from assessing his subjective quality of life in a reliable way due to cognitive, affective or reality oriented distortions (Katschnig, 1997).

The influence of symptoms is sometimes seen as a confounder, or something that has to be partialled out when analysing results of quality of life studies. Once psychopathology has been controlled, researchers can have a look at the associations of other variables of interest with perceived quality of life. On the other hand the domain of mental health is a vital part of a quality of life concept, especially within the field of psychiatry and the mentally ill. If subjectively perceived psychopathology has repeatedly been associated with subjective quality of life, perhaps researchers should include it in a more thorough way in a quality of life concept, rather than look upon it as a confounder. The findings of the Priebe et al., (1998b) study, investigating the interrelationships between subjective measures of needs, symptoms, quality of life and patient satisfaction, might speak in favour of this. In a factor analysis of these measures, a general factor explaining around 50% of the variance in the used instruments was found. This factor was loaded by variables relating to needs, quality of life and symptoms. Perhaps the content of this general factor should be explored with regard to an advancement of quality of life definitions within the field of the mentally ill. Obviously, there is a great overlap between perceived needs, subjective quality of life and perceived symptoms. The question is, how should it be interpreted?

Corten et al., (1994), in a study which aimed to develop a comprehensive model of subjective quality of life, found what they called a three-dimensional model where one of the dimensions, which they labelled hedonism, was strongly determined by a diagnosis of depression. Furthermore, Naess (1994) discussed the Polyanna syndrome, and the role of self-deception in the individual's perception of quality of life. In this paper she stated that there is empirical evidence that depressed persons are less characterized by self-deceit than non-depressed persons, and accordingly it would be the non-depressed person who exercises more distortion in the evaluation of subjective quality of life.

Psychopathology and quality of life are basically independent constructs, but the subject of their relationship deserves further discussion. In the advancement of such a discussion it is important to avoid a further blurring of the borders of the quality of life concept. A final comment on this subject is that the relationship between psychopathology and quality of life might not be resolved through cross-sectional studies, which has been the design of most studies discussing it so far. Longitudinal studies with a repeated measures design would throw more light on the causality and interactions over time of this relationship.

The relationship between subjective quality of life and other outcome measures

One of the conclusions from Lauer's review is that researchers should further investigate the relationship between subjective quality of life and other subjective satisfaction concepts and outcome measures, such as patient satisfaction. Like quality of life research, the area of patient satisfaction research has struggled with conceptual issues. It has been criticized for being vaguely defined, and has often been measured by *ad hoc* instrument, although there have been efforts to change this situation during the last decade (Ruggeri, 1994; Hansson, 1996). There has been a discussion parallel to that within the field of quality of life, concerning which domains or dimensions of services to include in measures of patient satisfaction. There has also been a discussion about the content validity of measures. This author has in the past advocated that measures of patient satisfaction should include dimensions of care and service delivery which are considered important by clients, and which reflect priorities from a client's perspective. Most measures in use have so far reflected the interests of information and priorities of service providers, which of course in a way is legitimate, but more in the context of quality assurance policies, than in a context of assessing patients' subjective experiences and satisfaction with services. One significant difference to quality of life research has been that there has been a much greater reliance on self-report measures.

So, what relationship is there between subjective quality of life and satisfaction with services? There are those who propose that satisfaction with services is not an independent construct; that it mainly measures general satisfaction with life or outcome of treatment, and not specifically satisfaction with services and interventions. A few studies have looked into the relationship of patient satisfaction and outcome of treatment, and most found that a better outcome is connected with better satisfaction with treatment. Subjective quality of life and patient satisfaction may also be related if viewed as process measures of an intervention. Patient satisfaction during various parts of treatment has been associated with compliance and participation in treatment, affecting progress and outcome (Office of Technology

Assessment, 1988; Bröker *et al.*, 1995). In a similar way, satisfaction with life and changes in it during treatment might be viewed as a broader process measure related to the course of treatment. Looking at it from this perspective, satisfaction with services and subjective quality of life are factors interacting with the course of treatment and the quality of patient–staff relationships in a service.

Lauer also concludes that quality of life should be related to other outcome measures. Obviously there have been, both in cross-sectional studies and in intervention studies, observed associations between quality of life and other outcomes, such as more narrowly measured clinical and social outcomes. One also has to remember that one of the reasons for developing quality of life measures was as a criticism against more traditional measures of outcome such as symptoms, functional status, etc., which did not capture the broader and more comprehensive interventions and outcomes aimed at in community-based psychiatric services. A second reason has been that quality of life used as an outcome measure would more appropriately reflect changes in the sickness panorama, with more people surviving illness, although maybe remaining chronically ill. So in order to be adequate, quality of life measures should tell us something more about people's lives than narrower traditional outcome measures. Whether quality of life should be viewed as a more general top-level outcome subsuming other outcomes is perhaps not primarily a conceptual question, but rather an empirical question which has not yet been settled.

Finally, Lauer suggests that researchers should relate quality of life to outcome measures such as readmission to hospital and community tenure. Since these are notoriously poor measures of outcome on an individual level, this would not add much to our understanding of the correlated outcome in terms of changes in quality of life. These measures are more related to availability of outpatient services, bed capacity and care policies than to the health and life situation of the client, and are therefore of less use in the context of quality of life (Hansson, 1996).

2

Methods for the assessment of quality of life in mental health care
WOLFGANG KAISER

Introduction

Some years ago an American methodologist, who had been asked to address a consensus conference on methods for assessing quality of life commented that his task was 'somewhat analogous to a General on the eve of a battle. The first task is to convince the troops that a battle plan is in hand. Once the battle begins, the second task was for the General to stay in front of the troops and provide some sense of direction to the events as they unfold' (Williams *et al.*, 1992). Continuing to use this same metaphor to describe the current situation in the field of mental health, it can be observed that considerable terrain has been captured during the 15 year period of quality of life orientated studies subsequent to Anthony Lehman's first studies (Lehman, 1983a; Lehman *et al.*, 1982). The issue which is now in question, is whether or not this position can be maintained – especially amidst signs of a rebellion and background opposition, and the longstanding phenomenon of scepticism about the validity and use of self-rating methods in psychiatry (Atkinson *et al.*, 1997; Barry and Zissi, 1997; Leimkühler and Müller, 1996). While the forces were advancing the methods used did not attract too much attention, but the question now is whether or not they have the capacity to keep the territory or even to advance further.

When considering methodological problems on the assessment of subjective quality of life, it is necessary to refer to the German quality of life instrument – the Berliner Lebensqualitätsprofil (BELP), to personal experiences as an interviewer of hundreds of patients suffering from chronic mental illness, and to a database of more than 2000 cases in which interviews were conducted using this instrument. Most of the following points could easily be applied to methodological questions relating to Lehman's Quality of Life Interview (QLI) (Lehman, 1988) and Oliver's Lancashire Quality of Life Profile (LQOLP) (Oliver, 1991a), also reviewed by both authors (Lehman, 1997; Oliver et al., 1997). The BELP is a close relative of the two quality of life interviews in the English language. Being a translation of the LQOLP it is a little shorter than the original and contains identical items; it also makes use of a Likert-type seven-point satisfaction scale to assess subjective quality of life, in the same way as its English counterparts.

Just like the majority of quality of life measures in medicine, these instruments have not been developed psychometrically in a laboratory – although a number of statistical tests have subsequently been carried out to produce some psychometric indices (Kaiser et al., 1996, 1997; Kaiser and Priebe, 1998; Lehman, 1997; Oliver et al., 1997). These quality of life measures have their historical background in the deinstitutionalization of long-term mentally ill patients and have been developed as an empirical approach to test and measure the humanistic goals associated with deinstitutionalization. Another slightly broader perspective would also suggest that these measures reflect the development of a more consumer-orientated approach to medical care in general, in which the patient's own opinion is awarded a much greater emphasis and importance (Gill and Feinstein, 1994).

This may explain why the construction of these instruments is so similar to indices which have been developed in medicine to measure such phenomena as severity of symptoms, functional disabilities, etc., by application of practical knowledge (Feinstein, 1987). Such 'clinimetric' instruments seem often to have more practical relevance and are more accepted than psychometric instruments resulting from laboratory work: 'Regardless of any disagreements on methodological issues, I think most scientists would immediately agree that clinimetric indices do have a very important humanistic value. The improvements shown with clinimetric indices are what most people seek in clinical care.' (Feinstein, 1987). The same seems to be true for quality of life measures and their value in the evaluation of psychiatric care. In this context, quality of life measures may also represent 'what most people nowadays look for in psychiatric care', a perspective which has emerged during the last two decades.

Although a narrow link with reform-orientated trends in psychiatry has to be acknowledged, psychometric criteria must have a clear priority as a frame of reference if an instrument is to be evaluated methodologically, even if it is subsequently considered in relative terms. These criteria have been developed during the history of the assessment of psychological constructs over nearly 100 years. They still serve as standards for empirical research in the field of mental health (Angst et al., 1991, 1994) as they define prerequisites for statistical methods adopted in all empirical studies undertaken using our instrument or its relatives.

Theoretical foundations

Campbell's remark from 20 years ago that 'quality of life is a vague and ethereal entity, that many people talk about, but which nobody clearly knows what to do about' (Campbell *et al.*, 1976) may now be considered to be a little outdated. Research in sociology and (social) psychology has led to a considerable body of empirical findings and a number of constructs or theories to explain well-being and satisfaction, for instance 'social comparisons' theory, 'adaptation level' theory or 'goal attainment' theory. For a review see Strack *et al.*, (1991).

Both in medicine and mental health, a distinction has to be drawn between generic and disease-specific quality of life models or constructs. The model behind, or rather the construct for, the BELP, LQOLP and QLI is a more generic one although these instruments have been mostly applied to people with severe mental health problems. It does not include the impact of psychotropic medication and psychopathological symptoms and related deficits, as Awad did in his more disease-specific approach in the field of mental health (Awad *et al.*, 1997).

Orley (Orley *et al.*, 1998) has used the confounding of dependent and independent variables in disease-specific instruments as a strong argument for the use of generic instruments: 'An instrument which focuses on assessing pain is not exploring the effect of pain on quality of life. Similarly, to assess the quality of life of a person with depressive illness requires an instrument that assesses all aspects of life, not just negative affect'. Another argument for the use of generic instruments is that they should be applicable across various diseases or conditions and to virtually everyone.

Satisfaction with pharmacological treatment, on the other hand, may play a prominent role in the life satisfaction of patients suffering from chronic mental illnesses, especially schizophrenia. When the question 'How satisfied are you with the effect of psychopharmacological treatment?' was included in a 14-item abbreviated version of the BELP in a carefully selected group of chronic DSM-IIIR schizophrenia patients, this item had the highest loading (0.85) on the first factor (47 variance) of a three-factor solution (varimax rotated principal components factor analysis). It may be useful to include disease-specific items as an optional module (and dependent variable) for different diseases in a general set of subjective quality of life.

Objectivity: interviewer biases

One of the difficulties with quality of life interviews using self-rating scales when carried out with chronically mentally ill patients is that very often it is not possible for them to make a clear choice of the satisfaction categories completely on their own. The ideal scenario in which the interviewer explains the satisfaction scale, then asks the question, after which the patient makes a decision, is not normally the reality. Very often questions have to be explained and the patient has to be assisted to make a choice between a 5-, 6- or 7-rating on the widely used seven-point satisfaction scale. The interviewer has to be careful not to influence the patient's response by his/her own interventions and bias. Even so, the varying mode of administration between patients depending on their ability to answer the satisfaction questions as self-rating in the mode of a questionnaire may be a source of potential direct influence on the ratings and may result in the introduction of bias in the study results (Aaronson, 1989).

The meaning which the patient attaches to the interview may be another source of indirect influence – although arguably this may also be true of many other assessments in psychiatry. For instance, the patient may fear that a high, or alternatively a low, quality of life may lead to the unwelcome termination of a placement in sheltered accommodation where he or she had hoped to stay for the rest of their life. Alternatively, the patient may assume that a low quality of life could lead to a report to their doctor who might then decide to increase neuroleptic dosage. Biases arising from the meaning attached to the interview by the interviewer may also be presumed. An example here might be where the patient's direct caregiver is also the interviewer. He might assume that if his client reports a low quality of life then it might cost him his job, or even, jeopardize the future of the whole project. The highly complex relationships between the caregiver and the patient must also be considered. From the patient's perspective, then, a low quality of life might either be suspected of leading to more intensive care, which may not be welcome, or alternatively it may be assumed to have the opposite effect. From the caregiver's perspective effects can also be hypothesized, e.g. does a low quality of life mean that he is not doing his job very well?

It is surprising, therefore, that no studies have been conducted to test interviewer bias in the assessment of subjective quality of life. Our own results (Kaiser et al., 1998a) in a random control study showed that the use of clinically responsible social workers as interviewers in sheltered living did in fact bias the interview results. Twenty-six interviews were compared and conducted by clinically responsible social workers with 26 others conducted by social workers from other providers who did not know the clients (clients were drawn and randomly assigned from a catchment area of 220 000 people). The mean score of the profile was significantly ($p < 0.05$) higher for the first group, indicating a higher satisfaction. All domains and general well-being for the first group also showed higher values. The mean difference for 'living situation' was statistically different ($p < 0.01$).

To come to this important and completely neglected point first, the answer concerning interviewer bias seems to be quite clear. There is absolutely no guarantee that either the interests or the assumptions of the interviewed people do not influence their answers in the sense of 'social desirability' or 'acquiescence'. The same is also true of interview style when the caregiver is also the interviewer. Clearly, further studies would have to be undertaken to test this question. So far the only solution for scientific work seems to be that the interviewers should be as independent as possible and that they should declare their neutrality and the protection of the interview data as explicitly as possible. These effects have to be taken into account in routine evaluation.

Other sources of interference

Psychopathological symptoms have an important influence on quality of life measures and a shared variance of up to 30% has been observed (Kaiser *et al.*, 1996, 1997; Lehman, 1983b). It could be debated as to whether or not these are actually features of the illness and a person's situation and therefore are partialled out statistically – as is often done in naturalistic cross-sectional studies with psychopathologically non-equal samples. Again this would refer to the objection of a confounding of dependent and independent variables. The solution may be to report both values, with and without controlling for psychopathological symptoms. It is necessary, however, to have a rating of psychopathological symptoms – usually the Brief Psychiatric Rating Scale (BPRS) – to make a decision at all. This rating should be undertaken by an independent rater since it could be speculated that broad information on a person's satisfaction might bias psychopathological ratings and vice versa. In routine evaluation it will often be difficult to have additional independent psychopathological ratings. This means, on the other hand, that the interviewer should not only to be experienced in interviewing patients with chronic mental illness but should also be trained in psychopathological ratings as well.

Almost all chronically mentally ill patients exhibit psychopathological symptoms to a greater or lesser extent, particularly those who are psychotic. Psychopathological symptoms do not affect the concept of subjective quality of life as a whole and can be discriminated as a separate construct (Kaiser *et al.*, 1996, 1997; Lehman, 1983). There is obviously, however, a level of acuteness above which any assessment of satisfaction is meaningless. This then raises the question of when to judge delusions or hallucinations as being beyond the limits of a useful interview. Even a rating of 'very mild' on the 'suspiciousness' item of the BPRS would imply that the patient is 'reluctant to respond to some "personal" questions' (Ventura *et al.*, 1993). More importantly, a 'moderate' rating should indicate verbal resistance and compliance only after rephrasing of questions. Inevitably this raises the issue of what the consequences are for the validity of a quality of life interview in these circumstances, even if one could be carried out at all.

Interestingly, our studies reported amazingly small numbers of patients who could not be interviewed in very chronic samples. It may be the case that more than 90% of the intended interviews were completed, but how reliable were the results? Obviously some criteria must have been applied to exclude some patients from being interviewed and it is therefore necessary to try to define and operationalize these. So far the only possible solution seems to be once again the conclusion that the interviewer should be clinically experienced and able to make a clear judgement.

Mental retardation plays a role among a considerable number of chronically mentally ill patients with a primary diagnosis of schizophrenia, personality disorder and others. While the influence of psychotic symptoms is examined in some studies (Kaiser *et al.*, 1996, 1997; Lehman, 1983b) the possible influence of mental retardation is neglected most of the time (Aaronson, 1989; Williams, 1991). Caregivers are often not able or willing to take this into consideration in general, possibly in the interests of 'political correctness', and thus the information about the proportion of mentally retarded patients in a sample is not very reliable.

In this author's experience, mentally retarded patients tend not to use the full scale, but will only give one positive and one negative response, often at the extremes of the scale. A numerable proportion of them in the sample (up to 20% in chronic patient samples) will lead to a further increase of ceiling or floor effects, produce a greater variance, and lead to more problems with the reliability of the results (or with the reliability of the reliability – concerning Cronbach's alpha: the value tends to approach 1.0 because mentally retarded interviewees perseverate and have a tendency to answer all questions the same way).

The influence of psychotropic medication on subjective quality of life is another possible source of interference in chronically mentally ill patients. Meltzer (Lehman, 1983b) used the Heinrich's quality of life scale in his study as an instrument. In the author's opinion this operationalized more of a deficit-syndrome construct than subjective quality of life, and demonstrated an effect of an atypical neuroleptic. Franz *et al.* (1997) and Awad *et al.* (1997a), however, demonstrated the same thing with different types of self-report methodology.

Neuroleptics can be hypothesized to have an impact in many different ways and additionally the response may differ between patients. A dosage which is too low should lead to an increased level of psychopathology. The same may be true for a patient who does not take the prescribed dosage. A dosage which is too high may lead to more inactivity and depressiveness. Apart from neuroleptics, antidepressant medication should also have an impact as may anticholinergics. A schizophrenic patient, who received a combination of a neuroleptic and an antidepressant substance, reported a significant change in her general well-being (3–5 on the seven-point scale) after a change in the antidepressant.

Scores

Sumscores or mean values across all domains as an overall measure have better psychometric properties (see below). The question arises, however, over which domain scores should be included. Some domains contain only a single item while others range up to four items. Furthermore, a significant number of patients do not meet the criteria to rate all questions. This applies to single as well as multiple-item domains. A person who lives alone, has no family or relatives and does not go to work simply cannot answer eight of the subjective questions, and this is a fairly typical situation for a chronically mentally ill patient. So if sumscores or mean values across all domains are used they should be calculated consistently for all subjects and domains, and items which have been included should be reported.

Another disadvantage of sumscores is that for a measurement of change in longitudinal studies different domains may be affected by an intervention in a different direction. For example, first admitted schizophrenics showed little (statistically not significant) positive change in most life domains within 9 months but this did not apply to the domains of leisure and social relations, where a negative direction of change was observed (Priebe et al., 1998b).

Profile coefficients like Cattell's r_p offer another opportunity to take all domain values into account concurrently. The similarity of complete profiles can be calculated. The problem is that similarity is rather high between different profiles (Kaiser et al., 1997). Apart from the problem of overall or single domain measures the use of mean values from Likert-type scales for group comparisons has important advantages. Covariates can be defined and partialled out by the use of analyses of variance with covariates. This can be important for naturalistic studies when comparing groups differing in a number of variables, which should be statistically under control. Cross-sectional comparisons between different samples of patients with schizophrenia, for instance, reduced differences after psychopathological scores were controlled to a considerable extent (Priebe et al., 1998b).

Percent values ('percentage of people satisfied') seem to have a good acceptance for the audience, although they can only be used for single items and the control of other variables of interest is more difficult or statistically impossible.

Reliability

The most important method of estimating reliability in the field of quality of life measures seems to be retest reliability regarded as a measure of stability (Cronbach, 1947), although few results supporting this have so far been published. It is obvious that a certain level of stability of quality of life measures has to be reached. For a scale with a very low stability it would not be possible to differentiate, for instance, between settings which are true relevant differences and those which just exist at the moment of assessment. The latter would probably differ from day to day because quality of life varies continuously.

It goes without saying that what is true for all retest reliability coefficients of other tests is even more true for those of quality of life interviews: a lot of them exist, depending on the intervals between the measures. This group thought that 4–6 weeks was a good interval to be tested for a group of schizophrenic outpatients (Kaiser and Priebe, 1996). At first glance, three coefficients (> 0.70) were considered to be acceptable:

1. The overall mean value: 0.86,
2. General well-being: 0.71, and
3. Finances: 0.84.

Others were not acceptable, or only acceptable with reservations. The stability for the 1.5 years interval was similar to that of normal people in the classic studies of quality of life from the 1970s and 1980s in the USA and West Germany (Campbell *et al.*, 1976; Glatzer and Zapf, 1984).

Retest reliability is also of significant importance for analysing single cases. A critical difference has to be defined between domains and repeated measures presumed to be significant and should be interpreted. This value, d_{crit}, is calculated in psychometrics by a formula, which includes the z value for a given probability of error (for $p < 0.05 = 1.96$), the standard deviation and the (mean) retest reliability of one or more tests (Lienert, 1969): $d_{crit} = z_{crit}\sigma \sqrt{2 (1 - r_{tt})}$. For differences in general well-being ($r_{tt} = 0.71$ and a presumed $\sigma = 1.5$) this would lead to $d_{crit} = 2.2$. Leisure ($r_{tt} = 0.45$) would have a $d_{crit} = 3$ and the sum-/meanscore ($r_{tt} = 0.86$) produces a $d_{crit} = 0.75$, which would be a difference of one point in the seven-point format.

General well-being and different domains should have a retest reliability of ≥ 0.75 to make solid use of single case application. This would make a significant difference of two points (σ presumed to be between 1.2 and 1.5). With reference to the sumscore (a $\sigma \leq 0.9$ in the 7-points format presumed) a retest reliability of ≥ 0.85 would be sufficient to make a one point significant difference ($p < 0.05$).

Internal consistency coefficients (usually Cronbach's coefficient alpha) show if all items/scales can be said to measure more or less the same and not completely different constructs which serves as another measure of reliability. If the values are too low it could indicate that it would make more sense to talk about work satisfaction, family satisfaction, etc., and no longer talk about quality of life and its domains. Whenever these coefficients are reported on from American, British or German studies they always range above 0.7. They are distinctly lower than those recommended for psychological tests but range at the lower edge of the psychometric criteria and seem to be sufficient (Nunally, 1978).

Wright and Feinstein (1992), among others, showed that a high internal consistency can lead to a low responsiveness to change and therefore values of a medium but sufficient size can be an advantage. To somewhat confuse the whole discussion, however, another German study (Moeller *et al.*, 1996) demonstrated a very good responsiveness to change for an instrument with an internal consistency of 0.96 while a second one demonstrated that three *ad hoc* developed rating scales led to a reliability of differences $[r_{dd} = (r_{tt} - r_{xy}) / (1 - r_{xy})]$ which was equivalent to the values of the Hamilton Depression Scale.

Sensitivity: responsiveness to change

There seem to be no reliable values which can predict responsiveness to change and psychometric properties of an instrument seem to be of limited significance (Aaronson, 1989; Williams, 1991). This means that it is necessary to test this issue directly by the use of repeated measures (pre-test and post-test) designs. The sample size which is needed to produce significant differences should be calculated in any case (defined effect, testpower) (Cohen, 1988) and may serve as an estimate of sensitivity itself (Oliver *et al.*, 1997).

Unfortunately there are only a very few studies using that design and the results differ (Barry and Zissi, 1997). A study from the UK (Barry and Crosby, 1996) showed very few variables to be sensitive to change. Our own unpublished results from our deinstitutionalization study did, however, differ and revealed a better potential to measure change. Overall, the number of studies in the field of mental health which tested the ability to measure change is small. A reason for differing results between these and other future studies might be that in addition another sort of responsiveness to change seems to exist. Quality of life seems to change over time without intervention, probably as a result of adaptation processes. In our cross-sectional studies (Kaiser *et al.*, 1996, 1997) the group observed a better quality of life for inpatients with a current hospital admission of more than two years compared to those with a stay of between 6 months and 2 years (other variables, including psychopathology, were equal). It could in fact make a difference for intervention studies if baseline measures are taken either after some months or years of an inpatient stay, or after another sort of exposure to a baseline setting. Our first admissions study (Priebe *et al.*, 1998b) demonstrated our lack of knowledge of change of quality of life in schizophrenia patients. This group had hypothesized that adaptation processes (including lowering of expectations) should lead to an improvement of subjective quality of life some time after first admission. After 9 months this did not prove to be the case. The group had to learn that any improvement, if it takes place at all, may be assumed to take place at later stages of the illness (but when?) and cannot be regarded as a simple one-dimensional increase after a low initial quality of life.

Validity

Although reliability is an important attribute, the most critical property of an assessment is its validity, or rather its validities. Criterion-related validity (concurrent validity and predictive validity) refers to defined criteria – presently existing or in the future. Discriminant validity demonstrates the opportunity to discriminate between groups of patients as well as related concepts whereas construct validity involves a more theoretical meaning and is not directly concerned with predicting a particular criterion (Cronbach and Meehl, 1955).

Concurrent validity, when defined as correlation to other quality of life measures, seems to be of limited interest. There is no gold standard which represents the ultimate norm, and measuring errors duplicate even if instruments are of the same type (assisted self-rating of what the patient says). Some information or hypotheses about different aspects of quality of life can be obtained but other aspects of validity seem to be much more important.

Predictive or prognostic validity is obviously one of the most interesting aspects of validity. Even psychopharmacological researchers formulated expectations in that direction: 'The quality of life assessment score may drop weeks or even months before symptomatological relapse and might perhaps be used to predict relapses' (Angst et al., 1991). These expectations seem somewhat naïve in the light of negative results in our own studies. The only study to date that has examined whether a criterion (rehospitalization) could be predicted by the patient's quality of life is that of Postrado and Lehman (1995). They discovered that rehospitalized patients differed in their satisfaction with family relations and that the satisfaction-with-family variable predicted rehospitalization within a 10 month period with an odds ratio of 0.8. Unfortunately, this is not too strong. The other problem is, as mentioned before, that a high number of chronically mentally ill patients have no contact with family members which meant that the other more useable domain values did not have a predictive value.

Discriminant validity could be demonstrated in different American, English and German studies. Results seem to be congruent:

- Psychopathological symptoms have a maximum of 30% shared variance (Kaiser et al., 1996, 1997; Lehman, 1983b) but they are independently associated with quality of life and are not part of the construct itself.

- Differences between diagnoses could be demonstrated (Barry and Zissi, 1997; Priebe *et al.*, 1998b) as well as differences between settings (Kaiser *et al.*, 1996, 1997).

Both latter findings are inconsistent and could not always be replicated. The lack of theoretical foundation and the small number of findings concerning construct validity are interconnected. More sophisticated ways of testing this 'postulated attribute of people, assumed to be reflected in test performance' (Cronbach and Meehl, 1955) have not been undertaken so far and the findings are restricted to factor analyses. In one of our studies (Kaiser *et al.*, 1997) the results among six groups of schizophrenics show three-factor solutions for two groups and two-factor solutions for the other. The percentage of variance for the first factor differs between patients with a shorter stay in hospital (although up to 2 years), long-term inpatients, and outpatient groups with long-term illness. Only few items/scales can be attributed to a general, overall structure of loadings.

Conclusions

Any user of an instrument should not only be enabled to recognize, but also to put a value on a specific instrument for clinical as well as for research orientated reasons. The sort of questions which can be examined by the use of the instrument, and what has to be taken into consideration when using it, should be clearly stated. In the opinion of the author the following guidelines can be formulated for the use of the BELP and similar instruments for assessing quality of life in mental health care:

1. The BELP does not yet have its foundations in a specific and elaborated theoretical construct of subjective quality of life. Findings from our own and other psychological and sociological studies suggest that it may be conceptualized as a dynamic result of complex psychological regulation processes.
2. Several illness and treatment related variables of influence should be under statistical control, especially when long-term mentally ill patients are examined for their quality of life: in particular, psychopathological symptoms and the most effective way to control them by psychopharmacological agents.
3. As long as no research criteria are defined to exclude patients with extreme psychopathology and mentally retarded patients, then judgement must be based on clinical experience and should refer to operational criteria as well. These should be reported and described in each study.
4. As the robustness of the interview against bias by direct involvement of the interviewers into treatment and caregiving has not been proved, interviewers should be as neutral as possible.

5. Quality of life measures should be used in cross-sectional studies when examining the effects of interventions in repeated measures (pre-test, post-test) designs. Prospective designs to test responsiveness to change and prognostic validity are of special interest.

6. Use in single case studies is possible if certain statistical criteria are respected.

7. It is desirable to increase the reliability of domain measures. The reliability of the overall mean score and the general well-being item seem to be sufficient.

2: Discussion

Advancing the methods for assessing quality of life

PETER HUXLEY

Introduction

This discussion follows the pattern of Wolfgang Kaiser's chapter and raises issues that seem to be profitable in terms of the improvement in methods for assessing quality of life. A good deal of the material presented here is based on work using the Lancashire Quality of Life Profile (LQOLP) in England and the USA, and on many discussions with workshop participants in London, Boulder, Manchester and Berlin.

Quality of life's clinimetric origins

Kaiser first raises the issue of the origin of the development of quality of life as a clinimetric rather than a psychometric development. This is an important point. Critics of the approach sometimes fail to recognize that quality of life is a multidimensional concept, and that, while some parts of the LQOLP were designed psychometrically, such as the affect-balance scale and the self-esteem scale, others were not. Looking at quality of life from the perspective of physical medicine, there has been a much longer tradition of attempting to reduce quality of life to a single score scale (Bowling, 1991). The idea of a single score has been resisted for two reasons. First, this is an oversimplification of the concept which results from assuming that quality of life is something akin to symptoms or intelligence, and secondly, one cannot add together the 'apples and pears' of the different life domains. The idea of a profile has been retained in order to maintain the distinction between the domains. This is a fundamentally important point, since clinicians, in particular, seem to treat quality of life in the same conceptual way as 'health' or 'illness'. There are, however, vast differences between the life domains, such as housing and social relationships for example, which make a simple summation meaningless.

Our reservations about the aggregation of items on the LQOLP apply more strongly to the 'objective' than to the 'subjective' ratings. In recent work, Davies and Huxley (1997), found that the aggregated mean score across the life domains behaves in exactly the same way as a global subjective well-being measure (for example Cantrill's ladder). That is, in a study of the three-month outcome of treatment of opiate-abusers in a primary care setting, improvements were significant on two global well-being measures, and the mean of the life domain subjective well-being scores (Davies and Huxley, 1997). Similar results have been reported elsewhere in this volume. In light of these results it is proposed that a more open-minded view of the possibility of an aggregated mean score be taken which reflects objective or material circumstances.

The desire to have a single score may also derive in part from the need to have an operationally acceptable and yet very simple measure. This tension about simplicity for operational purposes is around in quality of life service evaluation (other authors discuss this later) but this should not divert us entirely from the profile approach because individual interventions may produce change within individual domains if the intervention is a potent one.

A related criticism is that the instruments omit important considerations. The main area which the Dutch, French and French-Canadians feel is missing can be summed up as 'the meaning of life' rather than its quality. One could say that this is missing in two ways, first as a domain which is rather more than just spirituality, and the second as a rating within each domain of the significance of that domain in the life of the individual. The problem raised by Italian colleagues concerning the current exclusion of questions about subjective well-being in respect of sexual relations from the LQOLP should also not be forgotten.

Another point which some critics miss is that the LQOLP for example was created in part as an assessment instrument, designed to capture in a more standardized way those social aspects which have ceased to be assessed systematically in clinical practice in the UK at least (Huxley, 1993). The LQOLP was therefore, in Kaiser's terms, developed clinimetrically.

Theoretical origins

Kaiser next raises the issue of the theoretical origin of the concept (and other authors have already discussed this). He is right to say that there is not much agreement about this, and that this has measurement consequences, as Oliver *et al.* (1996) have pointed out. The main theoretical issue is where does one stop measuring quality of life and start measuring other things, such as needs, for example?

Priebe *et al.* (1998b) conclude that self-rated measures, of symptoms, needs, and quality of life are correlated, and one general factor accounts for 43–55% of the variance of each. The subjective assessment of treatment was not correlated with the other constructs. The group concluded that different measures of subjective opinions may be required for the planning of delivery of care and treatment. It is necessary to increase the variance specific to each measure in order to ensure that one is not measuring the same thing with different instruments.

Individual values

Rather than get the relative valuation of life domains, one should re-examine the underlying assumptions in some of the ratings, as was undertaken in Berlin. So, for example, there should be some way of assessing how an individual values going out socially, or talking with friends. Are these things of no consequence to them at all? Do they like to be on their own? If so, then they should be getting a good subjective score if they don't mix much socially and get a low objective score. To some extent this is removing some middle class norms from the instrument. In data from the UK700 case management trial, it was observed that positive and negative changes in circumstances are, by and large, associated with positive and negative changes in subjective well-being. For schizophrenia sufferers only, however, an increase in social contacts led to a lowering of well-being. For schizophrenia sufferers this is not a counterintuitive result, since the overstimulation they feel from social contacts contributes to withdrawal and relapse in certain cases.

By re-examining the individual questions which make up the sub-domain scores, it should be possible to avoid the problem of mixing up the direction (poles) of different items within each sub-scale or the mixing of items of a different order, for instance, what one does at home and what one does out of the home in terms of leisure.

The other area to be included is not motivation, but for the long-term group, lack of insight (Dickerson *et al.*, 1997). The lack of insight may be measured to see if it is an intervening variable (between objective and subjective well-being) for the most disabled or ill. Preliminary data from the UK700 case management trial suggests that insight does not affect objective–subjective relations (Evans, 1998).

Another approach that may be adopted is to do more with the restriction variables, i.e. those that ask an individual 'would you have liked to do more of this but could not for some reason?' It is unclear what area these questions tap into. In the Prism (1997) study, a significantly lower quality of life was found in those who had restrictions in leisure, living situation, legal and safety, family relations and health. Does this indicate greater need, lower social functioning, lack of insight or what? Perhaps it is necessary to unpack the social relationship variables more. Some of the questions in the social relationships section came from Weiss (1974). His view of social relationships is based on the idea that social relationships make provisions for people, and they can be categorized in terms of these provisions. These provisions are defined as attachment, social integration, nurturance, obtaining advice and guidance, reassurance of worth and a sense of reliable alliance. Patients may differ in the extent to which they wish to have these provisions filled, and their subjective well-being may vary accordingly.

Interview completion

Kaiser raises the problem of respondents who cannot complete the interview, and of interviewers who help them to do it. How many patient really cannot do it and need help? Maybe the rate reveals differences in the population. On the other hand the problem may be due to unwilling or untrained interviewers. The follow-up of the Huddersfield cases has over 90% (Knight, personal communication) whereas the follow-up rate in the Prism study was much lower. Twenty-five percent of the psychotic cases in the Prism study refused to participate. Refusals and those lost to follow-up are potentially major issues for service evaluation and the continuous or regular collection of data. This should also be addressed. One also needs to be careful when interpreting results where there are many missing data.

To use trained and independent interviewees is expensive for services. One solution might be to examine the reliability and validity of worker-administered quality of life measures compared with independent outsiders by using a routine audit procedure on a smaller number of the cases. When a large number of service interviewers is used, it is possible to identify those who produce 'deviant' results. Some interviewers are more likely to produce a change in the patient's global well-being rating between the beginning and the end of the interview than are others (Oliver et al., 1996). Kaiser (this volume) has suggested that the persons responsible for the care of the patient do have an effect on patient subjective ratings. This effect is stronger for ratings of satisfaction with services as one might expect. Kaiser argues that more attention should be paid to the meaning of the interview for both the interviewer and the respondent. There are a number of congruent issues that could be examined. Two examples are shown in Tables 1 and 2.

In Table 1 items A and D are unproblematic but what is going on in B and C? B may be due to a lack of insight on the part of the patient, or worker misjudgement. On the other hand, there is the possibility that B is due to the user wanting to reject help, and C to wanting to acquire more.

Table 1.   Congruence issues (i).

	Worker rates high QOL	Worker rates low QOL
User rates high QOL	A	B
User rates low QOL	C	D

Table 2.   Congruence issues (ii).

	High need	Low need
High QOL	A	B
Low QOL	C	D

The relative proportions in each cell may differ from study to study and this might enable us to throw more light on this issue. Missenden *et al.* (1996) found staff and patient groups' own quality of life differed objectively and on some but not all of the subjective ratings (self-esteem, mood, leisure, social relations and health). She also found that different variables predicted global well-being in the two groups. In the patient group objective freedom and satisfaction with health were the best predictors, whereas for the staff, satisfaction with living situation and negative affect and satisfaction with family were the best predictors. In a study comparing Casablanca (Morocco) with Portland (Oregon, USA), community controls in both places had superior quality of life. In terms of freedom from psychological distress, interpersonal interactions had a much more important effect in Morocco and independence a more important effect in Portland, and in both cases more highly rated in the control groups. In terms of overall psychological well-being basic needs satisfaction was most important to the Casablanca patients, normal controls and the Portland patients (but not to the Portland controls for whom social support and skills in the home were more important). This probably reflects the better level of basic needs provision in Oregon. Independence was important to the Casablanca controls (as was objective freedom in Missenden *et al.*, 1996) and the Portland patients.

In Table 2, B and C are not a problem but it is necessary to understand what is going on in A and D. If these ratings are made by the patient then some of the conditions Kaiser suggests may apply. If the need ratings are by the worker and the quality of life ratings by the patient (as is commonly the case), then A and D may be associated with patient lack of insight or poor worker assessment. On the other hand, A may be the user rejecting help, and D the user seeking more. Again, the relative proportions in each cell may differ by client group or study, and this may help us to explore what is happening. It may be that the influence of psychopathology is greater in some cells than in others. There is sufficiently consistent evidence now for us to accept the effect of depression on quality of life scores (Oliver *et al.*, 1996; Holloway, 1996b; Evans, 1998) and this should lead to the routine assessment of depression prior to quality of life assessment and perhaps to the exclusion of some cases, or at least a delayed quality of life assessment. Lack of insight has been assessed in the UK700 study, and while these data are still being analysed, preliminary results indicate that people who lack insight have significantly higher ratings of their subjective well-being with their own mental health than those who do have insight (Evans, personal communication).

The role of psychotropic medication

Researchers seem to know less about the role of psychotropic medication in quality of life assessment. The dose may not be adequate. In some places, the treatment consistency or quality remains unclear. Holloway (1996b) found that side-effects of medication were unrelated to quality of life unlike Sullivan *et al.* (1992) who found a correlation. In the Casablanca–Portland study, medication effectiveness may have accounted for the better quality of life of the Portland patients and for the fact that negative symptoms as opposed to the better-controlled positive symptoms were associated with a lower quality of life.

Scoring issues

Kaiser raises the problem of non-response in several quality of life domains because they do not apply to all respondents. The solution to this remains unknown. Perhaps using higher concept domains but fewer of them? As he points out, both means and the percentage which are satisfied are useful scoring methods but for different purposes. However, the importance of the profile concept and the distinction between what is a clinically meaningful difference and a statistical one should still be remembered. The individual patient is not interested in the extent that their improvement or deterioration was due to chance. Catell's r_p coefficient may be useful in analysing the results when expressed as a profile; perhaps researchers should be doing more with this measure.

In terms of the other issues raised about scoring, the following observations should be made. The stability of self-reported quality of life could change very quickly because of a major event; should the test–retest period therefore be shorter than weeks? (Kaiser and Priebe, 1998). Should the use of analogue scales be considered for the detection of change? (see below). It is the author's view that the coefficients for internal consistency compare favourably with other instruments in the field of social psychiatry.

Change over time

Kaiser addresses the question about responsiveness to change over time. A number of authors have argued that quality of life measures are relatively stable over time. Barry *et al.* for instance (1993) support this view. However, their original study only involved patients who had moved within the hospital. It is therefore not surprising that only the living situation ratings of the patients had changed. This suggests that targeted interventions are likely to produce changes in specific domains. Max Marshall (Prism Conference, 1997) shows quality of life unchanging over a period of time in his case management study, but he also shows that clinical symptoms were also unchanging, and this suggests that what researchers are looking at here is an example of an ineffectual intervention. Preliminary data from the UK700 case management trial show that objective quality of life changes in the lives of these severely ill patients were very limited.

Validity issues

Kaiser raises the fundamental question about validity – is quality of life measurement of any use and if so for what? As Kaiser states, there has been little work undertaken on predictive validity of quality of life measures. The current UK700 study will be able, eventually, to throw a lot of light onto this question. It is the author's impression that the discriminant validity results are fairly good and consistent; take, for example, the cross-cultural comparisons (Warner and Huxley, 1993; Warner and Girolamo, 1996; Heinze *et al.*, 1997). It also seems to be the case that inpatient and outpatient samples can be distinguished (Kaiser *et al.*, 1997; Prism Conference, 1997). There is also a consistency in the relationship with age and marital status; this has been observed repeatedly (Oliver *et al.*, 1996; Prism Conference, 1997) including in the so far unpublished UK700 study (Evans, personal communication). As one might expect, as one grows older, life satisfaction tends to increase, and the state of marriage is inherently more satisfying to men than to women!

3

The use of quality of life measures for service evaluation in mental health care

KARIN HOFFMANN

Introduction

In the last few years, service evaluation has been a growing issue in social psychiatry and public health. This trend is supported by the increasing number of publications (Becker, 1995; Bond et al., 1988; Borland et al., 1989; Hoult, 1986; Leff, 1993; McCarthy and Nelson, 1991; O'Driscoll, 1993; Okin et al., 1995; Thornicroft and Breakey, 1991). The interest in this field of research has been due to many different reasons some of which are scientific while others are of a more practical nature. Since the 1970s and 1980s, a system of psychiatric community care has developed and expanded. Community care systems incorporate a number of different services for treatment, day structure, occupation and sheltered accommodation. Changes in the structure of the psychiatric care system (especially the shift away from hospitals as a place of treatment to the community and the movement of deinstitutionalization) has led to a wider interest in service evaluation.

In Western Europe services have some similarities. However, there are some special conditions in Germany in contrast to other countries, for example England, which has a public health system. In Germany, the health care system is split into different kinds of providers and purchasers. It also employs different forms of financing. There are both public and private sector providers of public utility services. Purchasers of psychiatric care are health insurance companies, health authorities, communities and social welfare. Some services are paid for in a lump sum. Other purchasers obtain funds for each particular service and each action provided. Some services of the psychiatric care system such as sheltered accommodation are financed at a daily rate for each patient. This money pays for wages, rent, management and other requirements.

The psychiatric care system was not planned by a central governing body. Its expansion was dependent on the specific conditions found at various places. In the beginning, it was questionable whether the new services would operate effectively, reaching the patients they were supposed to. Subsequently, a practical and scientific interest was developed to determine the effects. Practitioners and researchers sought new findings on the consequences of specific programmes and treatments in an attempt to establish a better understanding of them. It was intended that this in the long term would help improve programme interventions. Corresponding to the fragmentation of the health care system, the view taken was very heterogeneous in nature. Staff wanted feedback on their own work as well as to secure their own posts. On the other hand, there was the economic interest of the providers who wanted to demonstrate – sometimes even legitimize – their work as being successful. The purchasers wanted to establish whether the services addressed the right clients and worked efficiently.

In other words, service evaluation always takes place in an area of conflict. Depending on the researcher and those being researched, there are specific interests and different goals. The same results of evaluation can lead to extremely different interpretations depending on the particular view of the various groups. Sometimes there are political interests and external pressures to obtain the 'right' or avoid the 'wrong' findings. In any case, service evaluation is thrown into a realm of different expectations from the viewpoints of politicians, practitioners, researchers, and other societal groups such as relatives and patients themselves. The researcher must be well aware of these conflicting interests and of his own task, otherwise he is in danger of being instrumentalized for the interests of a particular group. For this among many other reasons, some scientists think that service evaluation is not a true matter of science but of business or politics. In contrast, some practitioners are of the opinion that researchers only discover what they already knew.

Initially, this chapter will introduce some of the general implications and difficulties of service evaluation, which the concept of quality of life shares with other constructs. Secondly, it will describe some of the specific problems associated with the concept of quality of life in service evaluation. It will then set an example for common methodological difficulties and report some of the findings from the 'Berlin Deinstitutionalization Study' on the quality of life in different settings. Finally, these will be presented with a practical model for evaluation in so-called complementary services, i.e. sheltered accommodation and day care centres, which was originally planned for implementation in Berlin, but has not been realized.

General implications in service evaluation

The object of evaluation

The first question which needs to be discussed is: What shall be evaluated? In other words, what is the object of evaluation: a service, a type of service, or a programme? (Wittmann, 1985). The following definition of these terms can be made for our purpose:

- A service is the smallest organizational unit for psychiatric community care with certain goals, defined clients and occupational groups, usual activities and methods.
- A type of service is the totality of all services, which share common goals, actions, resources, underlying theories and certain programme elements.
- A programme is a specific kind of intervention that can take place in different types of services.

For example, a researcher is commissioned to evaluate day care centres. Does this mean the evaluation of the type of service? In other words, the evaluation of all day care centres in a given area, or the evaluation of a particular one? In the first instance, one can draw conclusions for the type of service, but not for a particular service. The researcher may discover that the examined day care centres operate very well. This however, would not necessarily apply to each specific day care centre. Alternatively, if the researcher evaluates an individual day care centre, the service can only be judged without drawing conclusions for the overall type of service. Let us suppose that the evaluation of a particular day care centre shows that it worked effectively. Obviously, there is no way of knowing whether there are special conditions in one specific centre. One example would be a highly motivated workforce – this being an essential prerequisite for the provision of a highly efficient service.

Conditions are in fact more complicated. Some day care centres offer patients a special programme, i.e. a psycho-education facility or a special kind of occupation such as the repair of bicycles or training of everyday skills. Each type of service can include different programme elements, and the same programme element can function as part of different types of service. It is therefore not possible to decide whether the finding that day care centres working well on average are caused by one specific element of the programme. For example, the successful work of day care centres may be due to occupational therapy, and only this element of therapy may produce the described positive effect. It would be wrong to assume, that it is the type of service (in our case the day care centre) which works very well. A day care centre without this special programme, i.e. without occupational therapy, would produce unfavourable results.

Usually, the object of evaluation research is a type of service or a programme and not a particular service. Most scientific publications in the field of evaluation examine a type of service. It must be recognized that each type of service constitutes several services with different programmes. There is no consensus when it comes to using the term 'service evaluation'. 'Service evaluation' is often used for both evaluating a type of service and evaluating a particular institution. It is in this context that the evaluation of the type of services will be considered.

The course of patients' characteristics and the quality of the service

It is a common procedure in outcome evaluation to draw conclusions from the course of certain patients' characteristics to the quality of a service, i.e. the quality of the therapeutic work. This procedure is often used in psychotherapy research where the criteria of outcome and parameters of treatment can be directly related to each other. It is not comparable to the field of community evaluation research. A service forms a setting which does not necessarily include the treatment as a whole. For example, a patient living in a therapeutic group home is treated by a psychiatrist who works in office practise and prescribes neuroleptics. Once a month, the patient consults with his social worker in the local health service. Occasionally, he may seek help from a crisis intervention team. Thus, the care a patient receives in a thera-peutic group home is only part of a comprehensive treatment and care package. Changes in the individual characteristics of a patient (such as the psychopathological symptoms or the subjective quality of life) can be influ-enced by interventions of all those who participate in the treatment. In addition, many known and unknown influencing variables exist (for example life's events) which cannot be comprehensively assessed or controlled. To conform to every element of the treatment package is therefore hardly possi-ble. Furthermore, a service cannot exactly define all parts of the treatment. There are no standard or generally accepted concepts for the care in thera-peutic group homes or day care centres. These concepts differ considerably from each other and are often not explicitly formulated. Thus, the explicit and concrete formulation of a treatment concept is the basic requirement for the evaluation of a service – a frequently neglected condition.

Small sample sizes

The utilization of quality of life data for evaluating mental health services shares the same problems with any sort of evaluative research that uses individual variables. A general difficulty in the field of mental health service evaluation is the small number of patients attending the same service. Services are often small. Some institutions for sheltered accommodation have just four patients. Most day care centres in Germany do not exceed more than 16–18 persons with 5–10 new admissions per year. Obviously, the usual statistical analyses are inappropriate for evaluating such small services because the size of the sample is too small. If one waited for 10 years to accumulate a suffi-cient sample size, there is the possibility that conditions of service and social circumstances may have changed with time. It would therefore be difficult to reasonably compile such data. Also, service planners cannot usually wait for a period of 10 years before evaluating a service. This seems a serious shortcoming in evaluative research, but, as mentioned above, this problem is not restricted to using quality of life measures.

Study design

In the evaluation of psychiatric services within the community, studies with a cross-sectional design are often used. These however, are not significant since the effect of the interventions and patient selection are confounded. For the purpose of service evaluation there is a need for longitudinal studies. For such longitudinal studies, many more financial and personal resources are required, although these occasionally border on the limits of what can be accepted by both patients and professionals.

Special implications for the use of quality of life in service evaluation

Levels of evaluation

On which level of evaluation can the concept of quality of life be used? (Abele and Becker, 1991; Baker and Intagliata, 1982; Gibbons and Butler, 1987; Huxley and Warner, 1992; Kaiser et al., 1996; Lauer and Stegmüller-Koenemund, 1994; Lehman, 1986; Oliver, 1991a; Oliver and Mohamad, 1992; Oliver et al., 1997; Postrado and Lehman, 1995; Simpson et al., 1989). In the discussion concerning quality management there is a commonly used distinction between the three levels: structure, process, and outcome.

- Structure level means the personal and local resources (staff, rooms, case-load, etc.) which are available as well as the general and the specific goals of this service;
- Process level refers to the way the interventions are carried out and monitored; and
- Outcome level means the effect and consequences of these interventions.

This distinction can be helpful for the following considerations. On which level can the concept of quality of life representing an individual character-istic of a patient for the purpose of service evaluation be used, and, secondly, on which level is it commonly used?

Structure

On the level of structure the following questions might be asked. Do the services care for the right people? Are the official goals congruent with the real conditions with regard to selection of patients? On this level certain elements of this concept can be applied – namely the objective variables – as a criterion for patient selection. For example, most services which take care of psychiatric patients in sheltered accommodation aim at looking after those patients who cannot live on their own without help, who have neither occupation nor day structure, who have no social net to support them sufficiently, and who need professional support in many everyday activities. The patients characterized above are possibly those with a poor quality of life. Do the services actually take care of those patients? Using an instrument to measure quality of life provides us with a clearer picture on patient selection and eligibility. Strictly speaking, some of the elements of the quality of life construct can be used, especially objective indicators for poor quality of life such as unemployment, homelessness, quantity of social contacts and long-term hospitalization, although this is not applied to the concept as a whole. The objective data used are very basic, not to say, trivial. One does not need the concept of quality of life to state these objective indices. It appears useless for this purpose.

Process

On the level of process it is the task of evaluation to examine whether the interventions are properly carried out and monitored. Applying the concept of quality of life on this level, one could observe whether there are specific interventions and support in particular domains of life to improve the objective and subjective quality of it. Furthermore, a service which periodically assesses the quality of life of its clients and regularly uses the concept for reflecting its approach, is provided with a good process quality.

Outcome

The concept of quality of life can also be used on the level of outcome evaluation which questions whether the service works successfully. With quality of life in mind, it could be asked: can the service improve quality of life, especially the general well-being or satisfaction with a certain domain? Indeed, one of the most important and most interesting questions, is how a patient's quality of life could be improved as an effect of interventions. To answer these questions it is not useful to conduct cross-sectional studies. Any interpretation of the findings to determine good quality of life will not identify whether it is the effect of effective care provided by the service or of patient selection, i.e. that the service selects only patients who already had quite a good quality of life before. Therefore, longitudinal studies are required to examine these types of questions.

What is a 'good' quality of life?

When using quality of life as an outcome criterion in evaluation, researchers have to remember the goal they are trying to achieve. At what level does the quality of life appear sufficient or at an optimum? These questions can be answered clearly for most of the other constructs used in evaluation.

The most established outcome criterion for evaluating psychiatric treatment is the assessment of psychopathological symptoms. Numerous scales have been developed, most of which have been used for evaluating short-term pharmacotherapeutic interventions. Psychopathology usually defines the illness. Thus, it is necessarily high and pathological at the beginning of the treatment. Treatment always aims at reducing psychopathology. Treatment aims at getting the degree of symptoms below a threshold that defines psychopathology. The optimal outcome is a psychopathological score of zero.

When subjective quality of life ratings are used for evaluation, the situation is less clear. There is no threshold below which a rating would be regarded as pathological. Scores may be lower than in the general population on average. There is however an overlap. Some patients are highly satisfied at the start of a given treatment; others may be entirely dissatisfied. Apart from the resulting floor and ceiling effects in cases of extreme values at both ends, the overlap with the general population at the beginning and end of treatment makes it more difficult to define the goal of treatment. Since patients with severe and chronic mental illnesses tend to be in services for a long time, the goal can hardly be that quality of life keeps improving all the time. When using subjective quality of life in the evaluation of mental health care services, scores of reference groups should be known and used for interpretation. While for most psychometric tests a comparison with the general population is sufficient, an interpretation of quality of life data requires more detailed and differentiated groups. Epidemiological data from the general population are required. Data from particular groups such as people who live alone, the unemployed and those on a low income are especially important. Quality of life data from patients in any service should be compared with data from such particular groups. Additionally, any service may build up its own reference group over time.

Sensitivity to change

To apply quality of life as a meaningful concept, i.e. as a criterion for evaluation in longitudinal studies, it must be assumed that the instruments employed are sensitive enough to assess changes over time. This has recently been questioned. In a study by Barry and Crosby (1996), a repeated measures design showed that after discharging patients from hospital, significant changes were evident in certain objective indices (living conditions, social contact and leisure activities), but only in one subjective index (increased satisfaction with living condition). This is not surprising, since it was the only domain that had really changed after discharging the patients. One could interpret this result as supporting the sensitivity of the instrument to assess specific changes. Measurable changes of quality of life seem to require very specific interventions. A recently published study (Kaiser and Priebe, 1998) used the Berliner Lebensqualitätsprofil and concluded that there was a good sensitivity to change regarding the general well-being and the sumscore of the profile. There is some evidence that an overall effect of interventions on quality of life (which in Germany is referred to as the 'water-can-effect') does not exist. Glatzer (1984) describes three different effects in subjective quality of life – generalization, compensation and neutralization. The results of Barry and Crosby (1996) seem to contradict the generalization theory but are consistent with the neutralization theory. Future studies are required to examine the different effects of well-defined interventions on the objective and subjective quality of life.

Validity

Many researchers have found and criticized that quality of life scores in severely mentally ill persons often lack face validity. This means that the results are not consistent with the expectations of the researchers and clinicians. Schizophrenia patients are frequently more satisfied with their life than one could expect from their poor objective living situation. They are not less satisfied than other groups with physical illnesses or social disadvantages, although they appear more disabled to researchers and clinicians. Patients in different services do not often differ in their satisfaction ratings, although such a difference would be consistent with 'common clinical sense'. These results have led some researchers to question the validity of the subjective quality of life ratings in the mentally ill. Thus, the lack of face validity is taken as the lack of any validity. This is, however, not an acceptable conclusion. It may well be that satisfaction ratings are not valid but for the time being there are alternative explanations. One may add that such a conclusion would be tautological: if face validity was defined by clinical impression, and if that face validity was crucial, the result of any sophisticated research could hardly be better than clinical impression.

Obviously, there is no external criterion for validity of subjective ratings. More qualitative research may test whether the results of rating scales are plausible in the light of detailed personal interviews. Nevertheless, for the time being researchers may have to live with the ratings they already have. However, the results should not be disqualified just because they are different from the expectation of those undertaking the research.

Quality of life: the adequate concept for service evaluation?

As explained in the beginning, service evaluation might sometimes adduce the 'wrong' findings. Why do some researchers and clinicians easily disqualify quality of life data that are not consistent with their assumptions? One reason might be that the failure to demonstrate a positive effect of services on patients' quality of life is a threatening result. Unlike other evaluation criteria such as the degree of symptoms, social skills, etc., quality of life may not be regarded as a 'run of the mill' evaluation criterion. It has the myth of being the ultimate criterion. What else remains to be achieved if there is no effect of the service on quality of life? Thus, negative results cast serious doubts on the usefulness of the examined service. If many services are found to have no effect on the patients' quality of life, it may be necessary to reconsider the rationale of our mental health care system, and of our researchers', and clinicians' qualifications and status. Quality of life research and, in particular, negative results, may pose a challenge to service evaluation and planning. On the other hand one could say that the concept of quality of life is too ambitious to be used in service evaluation. Perhaps using the concept of quality of life is also an expression of our efforts to do the best for our patients and to demonstrate our professional activities as effective. It is necessary to improve the living conditions within the community for the severely mentally ill. Patients should have more friends and leisure activities, improved living conditions, better physical and psychic health and, in general, greater satisfaction. Researchers may have to learn more modesty in their aims and expectations of what mental health services can achieve, or just confine those aims. With this view in mind, quality of life could be the wrong concept used to assess and evaluate mental health services. It then becomes necessary to further research and develop new ideas.

Findings from the Berlin deinstitutionalization study

Findings of the longitudinal Berlin Deinstitutionalization study (Hoffmann *et al.*, 1997, 1998; Kaiser *et al.*, 1998b; Priebe *et al.*, 1996), illustrated some of the methodological problems which may arise. This study evaluated the process of deinstitutionalization in three catchment areas of Berlin with approximately 550 000 inhabitants. It was an evaluation study under naturalistic conditions with a repeated measures design. The inclusion criteria involved a continual hospitalization time of at least 6 months and a place of residence before the last hospitalization in the catchment area. At the baseline, all patients were personally examined and interviewed. In the follow-up study, discharged patients were examined 1 year after resettlement within the community, whereas hospitalized patients were interviewed 1–2

Table I. Sample of patients in the Berlin
Deinstitutionalization Study.

N	142
Age (years)	47
Women (%)	44
Schizophrenia (%)	80
Affective disorder (%)	5
Addiction (%)	8
Other diagnoses (%)	7
Number of hospitalizations	9
Duration of hospitalization (years)	9
Psychopathological symptoms at baseline (BPRS)	44
Psychopathological symptoms at follow-up (BPRS)	41

years after the first interview. The instrument was the German version of the Lancashire Quality of Life Profile called the Berliner Lebensqualitätsprofil (BELP) (Kaiser and Priebe, 1998; Oliver *et al.*, 1997; Priebe *et al.*, 1995). Other instruments used in this study were the Brief Psychiatric Rating Scale (BPRS) (Overall and Gorham, 1962) to state the actual psychopathological symptoms, the Berliner Bedürfnis Inventar (BeBI) (Hoffmann and Priebe, 1996; Priebe *et al.*, 1995) for needs assessment and the Klientenbogen zur Behandlungsbewertung (KliBB) (Priebe *et al.*, 1995) for assessment of consumer satisfaction, a combined form of v.Zerssens Beschwerdenliste assessing subjective complaints, and a short form for the assessment of the physical needs of care. Besides these, some demographic and clinical data including diagnoses using the ICD 10 (Dilling *et al.*, 1991) were considered in addition to information about onset of illness, number and duration of hospitalizations.

The findings presented here include all data collected prior to September 1997. The question that was examined was: what is the course of quality of life in those patients affected by different types of service? Table 1 shows the sample of patients examined. The number of patients interviewed totalled 142 with a mean age of 47 years; 44% of them being female. The majority of patients were diagnosed with schizophrenia. The cumulative number of hospitalizations was approximately nine, with a hospitalization duration time of 9 years. Current psychopathological symptoms were seen to be moderately strong (mean sumscore of BPRS was 44 at baseline; 41 at follow-up).

Four groups of patients can be differentiated, as follows:

1. Hospitalized patients who stayed in the same hospital,
2. Hospitalized patients who had been transferred to another institution (hospital or hostel for psychiatric patients),
3. Discharged patients, who were hospitalized for less than 1 year or who had been returned to their own home (short-term/returner group), and

Table 2. Sample of interviewed patients differentiated into four groups.

	Hospitalized (same hospital)	Hospitalized (elsewhere)	Discharged (short-term/ returner)	Discharged (long-term hospitalized)
N	63	14	21	44
Age***	54	50	47	42
Gender (female)*	43%	43%	62%	25%
Diagnoses:				
Schizophrenia	94%	93%	57%	66%
Affective disorders	0%	0%	19%	7%
Addiction	2%	7%	19%	14%
Other diagnoses	5%	0%	5%	14%
Number of hospitalizations	10	7	12	8
Duration of hospitalization***	185	49	27	73
Psychopathology***	47	42	33	36

*p < 0.05; ***, p < 0.001.

4. Discharged patients with hospitalization duration of more than 1 year (long-term group).

Group four can be referred to as the 'true' long-term patients. In most cases, these patients are discharged to sheltered accommodation. Table 2 shows data for these four groups. There are many significant differences between the groups. The discharged long-term group is significantly younger than the other groups and there is only a low percentage of females. About two-thirds of these patients are schizophrenics when compared with 93–94% of the hospitalized groups. Their psychopathological symptomatology (mean 36) is not very high.

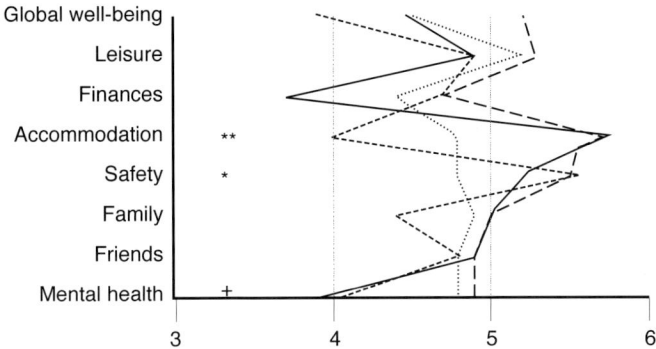

Figure 1. Subjective quality of life in four groups of psychiatric patients
Key: •••• Hospitalized patients (same hospital), – – – Hospitalized patients (in another hospital/hostel), —— Discharged patients (short-term), — — Discharged patients (long-term). ⁺p<0.1, *p<0.05, **p<0.01.

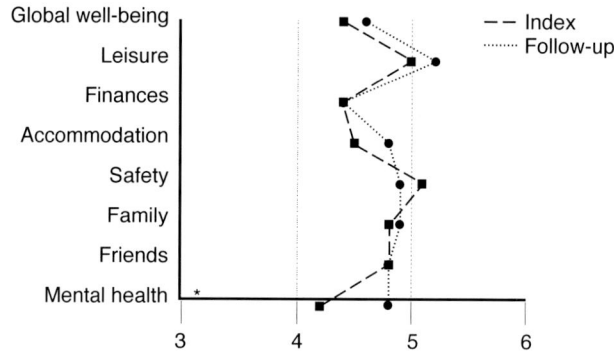

Figure 2. Changes in subjective quality of life in patients hospitalized at the same institution. *p<0.05.

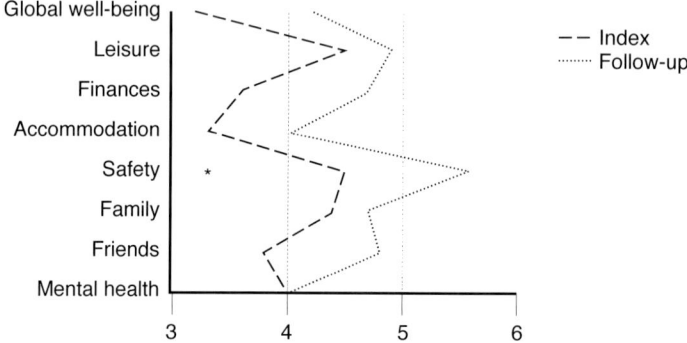

Figure 3. Changes in quality of life in patients hospitalized elsewhere. *p<0.05.

When comparing profiles of subjective quality of life cross-sectionally (see Figure 1), some clear differences can be recognized. In general, the profiles of both discharged groups show higher satisfaction; the differences are significant in the domains of accommodation and safety. Surprisingly, findings show that those patients, who were hospitalized in another institution, stated the highest satisfaction in the domain of personal safety. As a result of the cross-sectional design, it remains unconfirmed whether the better quality of life of the discharged patients was a result of a specific setting or whether these patients actually had a better quality of life in the beginning.

Figures 2–5 show the changes in profiles of subjective quality of life for the four groups between baseline and follow-up stages. Those patients who stayed hospitalized in the same institution (Figure 2) showed no changes in satisfaction other than an increased satisfaction with mental health. The profiles appear to be very similar. Those patients who were transferred to

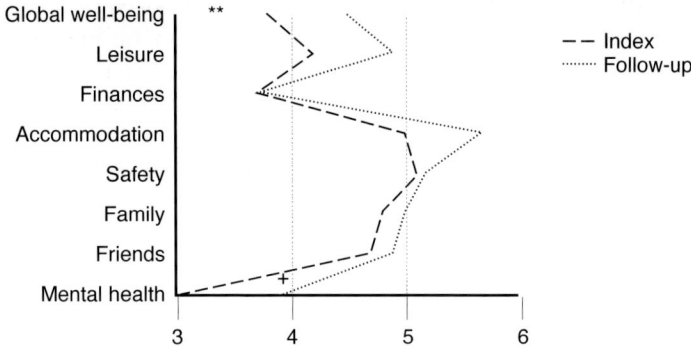

Figure 4. Changes in subjective quality of life of discharged patients (short-term/return-ers). **p<0.01, +p<0.10.

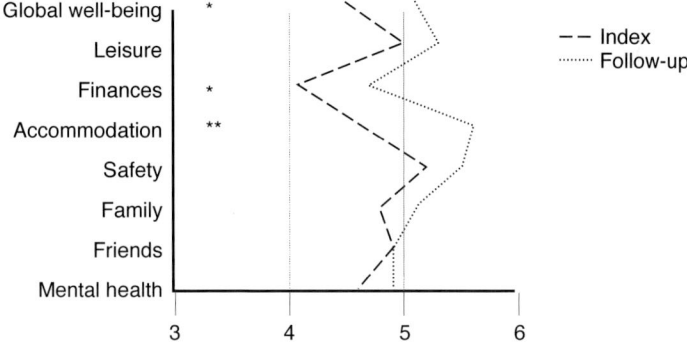

Figure 5. Changes in subjective quality of life of discharged patients (long-term hospital-ized group). *p<0.05, **p<0.01.

another hospital or hostel (Figure 3) stated significantly higher satisfaction with their safety. The course of the profiles is nearly parallel. The discharged short-term group (Figure 4) shows significant changes in their satisfaction regarding general well-being. Most changes are shown in the discharged long-term group of patients (see Figure 5). There is no significant negative change. Significant changes can be seen in the general well-being and in the domains of accommodation and finances.

What kind of conclusions can be drawn from these findings? It can be seen that the discharged long-term patients have the greatest change in their satisfaction in comparison to other groups. As a rule, these patients live in sheltered accommodation. Does this mean that these services work well? The results can provide us some reference to this conclusion but do not prove it. Some limitations must be recognized:

- The study did not incorporate a random controlled trial. It may therefore seem possible, or likely, that there is a systematic bias of patients' selection for the different settings. It can be seen that the age group of the long-term discharged patients was younger than the other groups. Maybe these patients are more likely to alter themselves in general.
- There were some drop-outs, but these patients may have had a lower quality of life.
- This group evaluated the type of service and not a particular service. Because of the small number of patients living within the same service, it was not possible to verify findings using the usual statistical procedure. It is not ethical to pass judgement on the quality of particular services. It still remains unclear which particular service works well or which one is ineffective. A last restriction was the fact that the samples were rather small and the number of patients in the different groups varied substantially.

In summary, the limitations described above mean that the results can only provide us with a cautious interpretation.

Is it possible to generalize these findings across Berlin, i.e. from the Western to Eastern part, from innercity districts to suburban districts, from rich to poor, and so on? It is unlikely that these findings relate to other cities in Germany. In Berlin, the conditions of sheltered accommodation concerning staff or case-loads are unique. Results cannot be transferred to districts with poorer case-loads. Even if they can be related to other large cities, results can hardly be transferred from city to rural areas. On average, patients in sheltered accommodation had a better quality of life than patients in other types of services. It is uncertain which specific elements of the programme – therapeutic setting or atmosphere – were responsible for the better quality. The findings are popular among the providers of sheltered accommodation and the politicians who support deinstitutionalization, or at least wish to reduce hospital beds in the hope of saving expenses; they are less popular among the advocates of hospitals.

A new concept for basic documentation and evaluation

Finally, this chapter will present a concept for basic documentation and evaluation as part of a quality management in mental health care services. This combines ideas about the structural framework of evaluation, its goals and thoughts regarding possible customers, concrete procedure, clinical and general purpose.

The starting point was the consideration that there are various 'customers' for evaluation each with different interests.

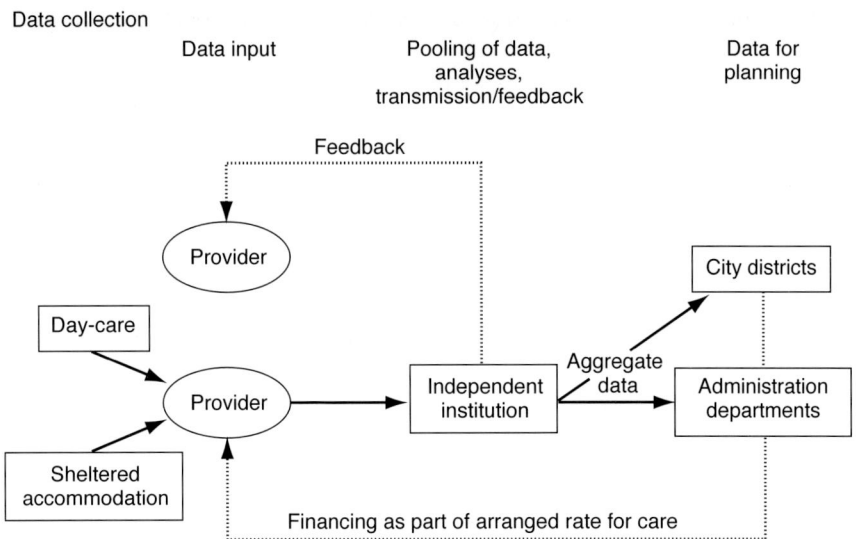

Figure 6. Model for documentation and evaluation in mental health services: cooperation contract.

- Staff members require feedback from their daily work and want to judge the patient's course,
- Service providers wish to demonstrate the effectiveness of the service,
- Patients and relatives wish to know what clinical practices occurred while the patient was in care,
- Administration departments need data as a background for planning and health reporting, and
- Sick-funds and other cost units are interested in a comparison of costs and utility.

In order to offer the various groups the specific data they require and are entitled to receive, a central independent institution is needed. Functions of this institution would include the pooling, analysing, anonymity of and transmission of data to various prospective customers, thus providing them with appropriate reference values (see Figure 6).

Mental health service evaluation has to consider several aims and principles. It must be comparable with existing systems of documentation, useful to all participants and practicable for the daily working environment. Therefore, basic documentation must be linked to evaluation and as a rule, data collection should be done by staff members. The quality of the data directly depends on the motivation of the individuals collecting it. Therefore, the members of staff must perform the interviews. However, there is a true dilemma because of the specific interviewer effect (Kaiser *et al.*, 1998a). Ratings of patients in sheltered accommodation will be more positive when they are interviewed by their own carers. On the other hand, when patients are asked questions by an independent interviewer and are assured of absolute confidence and discretion, data cannot be reported back to the personal carers. The main advantage with this model, i.e. evaluation as a module of quality management is not ensured. For this reason, the loss of the interviewer's independence is a necessary evil, which cannot be avoided.

Staff members see the concept of quality of life as being relevant. In contrast to the psychopathology which is only of small practical use, quality of life has immediate relevance for practice. Individual treatment planning can be connected with the quality of life interview. The staff can get feedback from their patients and can find out which life domains need improvement. Furthermore, staff get to know to what extent patients are satisfied or dissatisfied with their different life domains, or in general. Last of all, service evaluation should not be an ongoing task and occupation for researchers without practical consequences. Service evaluation must not become *l'art pour l'art*. If staff notice poor objective or subjective quality of life in particular domains of life, it should stimulate change in their current interventions or the development of new interventions. For example, a patient in a group home is very dissatisfied with his occupational situation, as a consequence, the staff can begin to search for a suitable occupation or a workplace with appropriate requirements. So the concept of quality of life can help staff to develop specific interventions in particular life domains. Employing the concept of quality of life for individual treatment planning is quite clear.

Likewise, the use of the concept is clear for service planning (refer to the example above). If many patients in sheltered accommodation are dissatisfied with their occupational situation a need for new services for these patients could be stated. Perhaps a new project should be started. Indeed, this happened in our own community care system. Many patients living in group homes had a poor daily routine and no occupation. For that reason, a small workshop for repairing bicycles was opened. On a larger scale, service planners who have data about quality of life at their disposal can draw conclusions about the existing services and for the development of new services. In summary, the advantages of the proposed model are:

- The longitudinal recording allows a clinical assessment and monitoring of the patient's course.
- Staff can periodically receive feedback on their work;
- Protection of data is ensured,
- It enables the researcher to evaluate the type of services,
- Data collected can also be used for planning and health reporting, and
- Data collection provides a basis for quality management.

This model of mental health service evaluation can combine three different functions: (i) individual monitoring of the patient's course, (ii) service assessment, and (iii) type of service evaluation. Despite these advantages, our model has not been realised in Berlin yet because of the many different fears of the providers concerning the transparency and the possible conclusions that could be drawn from the findings.

Conclusions

1. It makes sense to perform regular longitudinal assessment of quality of life as a matter of routine. The benefits are clear regarding individual monitoring and service assessment.
2. The results cannot be analysed by the usual statistical procedures.
3. It is necessary to improve the framework for interpretation and to build up reference groups step by step.
4. Evaluation of the type of services is an ongoing task.
5. Assessment and evaluation must be integrated into a comprehensive quality management.

I would like to finish with a quotation of a well known evaluation researcher (Rossi et al., 1988) who writes: 'In a nearly perfect world, where everyone can live in best health for many years, where there is no crime but social justice, where there are rich possibilities for occupation and social participation, where the existing social programmes effectively and efficiently solve the individual, social, and community problems, one would rarely do evaluation. Neither would there be a need for new programmes, nor a need for modification of existing programmes; and established programmes would not have to be supervised. Therefore, evaluation is the expression of our efforts to create a better world.'

3: Discussion

Quality of life evaluation in health services research

IAN DALY

Approaches to evaluation of health services

Health services can be evaluated through the analysis of model treatments or interventions or through programme-level research. Randomized controlled trials represent the 'gold standard' ensuring, as they do, greater internal validity; that is, that the hypothesized treatment effect is an actual consequence of the intervention. For these reasons, the most influential type of health services research is likely to be the experimental evaluation of model programmes or interventions. As will be seen in the next section, established quality of life measures have had relatively little application in this area and have therefore yet to prove themselves as robust or reliable indicators of outcome. Observational or quasi-experimental designs are typical of programme-level research which addresses the ongoing activity or operation of services and is conducted within naturalistic settings. It is primarily within studies of this nature that quality of life measures have been introduced over the past two decades.

Quality of life as an outcome measure

Health outcomes were traditionally measured using rather crude indicators such as mortality or hospital admission rates. Alternatively, service inputs or processes were themselves used as proxy outcome indicators, quality being equated with the range and availability of these inputs. Over the past two decades, however, and particularly as part of the ongoing assessment of community treatment programmes, increased reliance has been placed on the direct measurement of a widening range of outcome criteria within a multiplicity of domains (Dickerson, 1997). Quality of life measurement is increasingly likely to be conducted as part of this broad assessment strategy in the evaluation of health services.

Gotay and colleagues have proposed a classification of end points when quality of life measurement becomes relevant in general medicine: when people are very seriously ill with incurable disease, when alternative treatments bring about otherwise equivocal results, when the benefit of a treatment that is more efficacious, say, for survival, is offset by deterioration in quality of life, and when a long-term determinant of treatment choice must be made because overall failure rates remain high even when interventions differ in their short-term efficacy (Gotay *et al.*, 1992). These end points may be largely transposed to psychiatric practice where long-term illness is often associated with pervasive disability and with incomplete response to treatments which may themselves have disabling side-effects. Baker and Intagliata (1982) produce further reasons to measure quality of life. It often makes sense to measure comfort rather than cure; complex programmes require complex outcome measures; it keeps consumer interest foremost; there is increased interest in a holistic perspective, and 'quality of life' is good politically.

Quality of life measures in health services research

Although schedules that measure various aspects of social functioning and satisfaction were developed earlier, quality of life instrumentation as such may be dated to the beginning of the last decade, with publications outlining the use of the Quality of Life Interview (QLI, Lehman *et al.*, 1982), the Oregon Quality of Life Questionnaire (OQLQ, Bigelow *et al.*, 1982) and the Satisfaction with Life Domains Scale (SLDS, Baker and Intagliata, 1982). In this review, studies which either introduced quality of life instruments or used them as principal investigatory tools to assess the life conditions of particular groups of patients will be presented first. They include descriptions of residential care and community aftercare programmes, comparisons of the quality of life of patients who are homeless or in residential care, and some day treatment and psycho-education programmes. Thereafter, studies of model treatment programmes, mostly assertive community treatment or intensive case management programmes will be described. In the latter studies, quality of life is usually one of a series of outcome measures designed to assess service effectiveness. Throughout all of these studies comprising quality of life measurement, only a small number have utilized both controlled designs and well-validated quality of life instruments, and they will be described in greater detail.

Studies introducing quality of life instruments in health services research

The Quality of Life Interview (Lehman, 1988) was first used to enquire into the well-being of patients discharged into community accommodation. The

QLI provided useful information about life factors, mostly in the social domain, which contributed to respondent satisfaction; in evaluating subjective and objective dimensions of quality of life, it demonstrated correlations between them which, however, were low enough to suggest that each measured rather different aspects of quality of life. It allowed the authors to bring attention to hitherto poorly recognized issues such as personal safety, and to suggest strategies for improving quality of life that went beyond simple quantitative provision but sought to match such provision to patients' perceived needs. In a subsequent comparison study of hospital and community residential patients, Lehman and colleagues (1986) noted that when demographic, clinical characteristics and objective quality of life conditions were adjusted for in the analysis, then the treatment setting had no significant independent effect on life satisfaction ratings. Simpson et al. (1989) used the QLI in a small study comparing hospital and community residents, and reported findings broadly consistent with those of Lehman, thereby providing further independent validation of the QLI. Levitt et al. (1990) extended the QLI by adding 'self-fulfilment' and 'adult education' sections and modified the 'living situation' section in order to apply the QLI to a study of patients in day treatment. Sullivan et al. (1991), in a follow-up study of discharged patients using the QLI, noted high rates of personal satisfaction in most life domains despite objective conditions of considerable poverty. In a further study using the QLI, Lehman et al. (1995a) compared 106 homeless with 146 domiciled persons, all with serious mental illness. While finding improved quality of life ratings across a number of domains, the authors noted that differences were not reflected in general life satisfaction ratings which did not differ significantly between the groups. Barry and Crosby (1996) reported the use of the QLI in a repeated measures longitudinal design study. Despite finding significant improvements on a number of objective quality of life indices, the authors found that subjective quality of life improved in only one domain – living situation – and commented on possible insensitivity to change of life satisfaction ratings.

The Lancashire Quality of Life Profile (Oliver, 1991a) is based on the QLI with certain modifications to reflect cultural variation and to accommodate multidisciplinary service-based evaluation of quality of life. Oliver and Mohamad (1992) used the LQOLP to compare the well-being of residents in different types of community accommodation but found no significant differences. Shepherd et al. (1996) used the LQOLP to compare the quality of life of patients in hospital and in a range of community residences, and their results were broadly consistent with previous studies. Difficulties in completing interviews by some more seriously ill patients led the authors to question the suitability of these relatively complex and lengthy instruments for such patient groups. Hoffmann et al. (1998) used the German version of the LQOLP, the Berliner Lebensqualitätsprofil (Priebe et al., 1995) in a pre- post-test design to compare groups of discharged and undischarged patients. In contrast to the findings of Barry and Crosby (1996), this study demonstrated greater responsivity of life satisfaction to changes in environmental status.

The Oregon Quality of Life Questionnaire (Bigelow *et al.*, 1982) was shown by Bigelow and colleagues (1991) to discriminate between patient populations and the general population, and also between groups of patients with different mental health needs, including chronically mentally ill patients, general psychiatric patients, and those with alcohol problems or with other substance abuse problems. Baker and Intagliata (1982) developed the Satisfaction with Life Domains Scale (SLDS) and, in a study of a community support programmes, reported findings similar to those of other studies, notably, high levels of respondent satisfaction which seemed at variance with lives which were often characterized by extreme isolation. Pinkney and colleagues (1991) used the client Quality of Life Interview (Mulkern *et al.*, 1986) to report on quality of life following participation in a rehabilitation programme and also reported a tendency to predominantly positive responses in subjective well-being. Skantze *et al.* (1992) used the Quality of Life Self-Assessment (QLS-100) inventory to assess how standard of living in a group of schizophrenic outpatients, which was comparable to that in the general population, would impact on subjective quality of life. They found that subjective perceptions of quality of life appeared to be independent of standard of living, and that 'inner experiences' represented one quality of life domain frequently reported as unsatisfactory.

General findings from studies

These studies, as a group, were exploratory, descriptive studies designed to evaluate the instruments as much as to describe the quality of life of patients using particular health service provisions. The instruments range from those such as the Client Quality of Life Interview (CQLI) which are mainly checklists whose items have not been developed into scales to those such as the QLI and the LQOLP which have been extensively evaluated on psychometric properties. Some general findings from the studies are summarized below.

1.   Discharged patients generally report greater quality of life than either the long-term hospitalized or the homeless. In the absence of controlled designs, caution must be exercised in attributing this better quality of life to environmental rather than clinically pertinent factors such as symptomatology for instance, which is a robust predictor of subjective quality of life (Kaiser *et al.*, 1997).
2.   Seriously mentally ill patients in the community frequently live in situations of considerable financial hardship, and are often lonely and isolated. Finances, in particular, tend to be rated lower than most other

domains. Dissatisfaction with health is another important concern. Personal safety emerges as a more important issue for respondents than might have been recognized previously. Concerns about personal safety seem to be of greater relevance for hospital rather than for hostel patients.

3. Despite these considerable environmental disadvantages, the satisfaction scores of discharged community residents are often disproportionately high in comparison to actual life conditions, and ratings of dissatisfaction are made relatively infrequently. It is not clear from the studies whether these findings represent a response bias, a regression to mean effect, a resignation response to long-term adversity, or some more inherent illness-specific factor.

4. The quality of residential accommodation is the objective condition that seems to make the largest contribution to higher quality of life ratings. Comfort, privacy, freedom of choice and personal control and autonomy are the factors most clearly identified with improved satisfaction ratings.

5. In general, satisfaction scores have only moderate correlations, at best, with social functioning or objective quality of life conditions. Some but not full correlation may suggest, as Lehman has indicated, a real value in having separate objective and subjective ratings since they seem to measure different aspects of quality of life. However, correlations are often too low or inconsistent, and this raises questions both about the validity of the scales as presently constructed and their usefulness as measures of effectiveness of certain social and clinical interventions. Further knowledge is required about various mediational factors which may influence the appraisal process by which patients with serious mental illness evaluate their life circumstances (Atkinson et al., 1997; Katschnig, 1997; Zissi et al., 1998).

6. The general life satisfaction measure approximates most closely to a single rating that represents quality of life as primarily conceptualized in these studies, that is, through a subjective perspective. This rating, however, seems, on occasion, to have little ability to effectively discriminate between different groups. The two longitudinal studies in the series produced conflicting results in relation to responsiveness to change of life satisfaction scores. Despite the encouraging results from the Berlin study, there remains a concern that life satisfaction, as measured in these studies, may have poor discriminant potential to reflect changes between groups or over time.

7. Finally, some studies have reported considerable difficulties utilizing these self-report methods within more seriously mentally ill groups. Some have responded to this by simplifying the self-report versions (Bigelow et al., 1990), others by advocating the use of external supplementary ratings (Katschnig, 1997). Quite where this latter strategy fits within a

concept of quality of life that seems to be dominated by the subjective perspective, as indicated by these instruments, is another question.

Studies of treatment programmes using quality of life measures

Following on from the ground-breaking work of Stein and Test (1980), a number of assertive community treatment (ACT) replication studies have been published. Most such studies tend to have their own adaptations and modifications including various forms of intensive case management (ICM). The most singular difference between the two is that where ACT studies provide intensive outreach care on a team basis, in ICM, one therapist becomes primarily responsible for the comprehensive care of usually about 10–12 patients. Case management, in turn, can be seen to adopt a broker-age model where the therapist becomes responsible for organizing access to treatments and entitlements, or a clinical case management model where greater emphasis is placed on direct therapeutic interventions from the thera-pist. Studies will be summarized under separate ACT and ICM headings, and randomized controlled studies using validated quality of life measures will be described first.

Random allocation studies of ACT programmes

Stein and Test (1980) developed the Community Adjustment Form (CAF) to assess life satisfaction, self-esteem and other functional outcomes in a randomized prospective study (N=130) of an assertive community treatment programme in Wisconsin. The CAF consists of 140 items covering areas such as leisure activities, living situation, employment, income, food and housing, family and social contacts, legal problems, medical care and agency utiliza-tion, in addition to self-esteem and life satisfaction (21 items). No psycho-metric data have been reported for the CAF. In addition to reducing hospital bed occupancy, the experimental group reported significant improvements in life satisfaction and also more employment, greater earnings for those who had obtained competitive employment, and more contact with trusted friends at one-year follow-up. Thereafter, following withdrawal of the experimental treatment condition, most gains including life satisfaction were lost by two-year follow-up. Interestingly, measures of self-esteem differed significantly at baseline, in favour of the experimental group. The authors suggested that this difference may have reflected the timing of self-esteem data collection which occurred a few days into the study at which time subjects in the exper-imental group were out of hospital while control subjects remained in hospi-tal. Subsequent evaluations through the study period revealed no difference between experimental and control subjects on measures of self-esteem.

In Chandler *et al.*'s (1996) large two-site (one urban, one rural) study, 252 patients with serious mental illness, were randomly assigned to an integrated ACT programme or standard care. The QLI was used to measure quality of life. Twelve month outcomes have been reported indicating no quality of life gains. Most other indicators of social functioning also showed no difference between ACT and standard-care patients. Employment was increased and less time was spent in hospital by the experimental group, but hospitalization rates were not significantly different. Three-year outcomes from this study will be of interest to determine whether the present results are confirmed, or whether social outcome tends to show measurable improvement only after a delay period (Wykes, 1994).

Lehman *et al.* (1997) conducted a randomized trial ($N = 152$) of ACT for homeless persons with severe mental illness. The ACT programme subjects were more stably housed, used fewer crisis services and were more regular attenders at psychiatric and substance abuse outpatient clinics. They showed significant reductions in symptoms and hospitalization over the 12-month follow-up period. On quality of life, both groups showed significant gains over the year, the ACT subjects achieving greater improvements in life satisfaction and perceived health status. Work and interpersonal relationships showed no differences between the groups. The study was somewhat limited by the relatively short follow-up period, the inclusion of a greater number of African–Americans in the comparison group and the availability of an increasing number of housing and clinical interventions to the comparison group which occurred during the time period of the study, and which presumably explained the significant improvements in symptom levels and quality of life scores for both groups over the year.

In a study of ACT at three community mental health centres, Bond *et al.* (1988) found that the ACT group spent less time in hospital in two of the three sites and otherwise showed no differences as regards medication compliance or quality of life. A disadvantage of this study was the existence of significant differences between the sites in the design of their programmes, thus reducing comparability in outcome across the groups.

In a small study of 35 patients randomly allocated to ACT or standard care, Jerrell and Hu (1989) found no differences on any outcome measures between the groups. Results may have been compromised by the small numbers involved and the fact that some control subjects had received case management services.

In a controlled study examining the effects of the Threshold Bridge Programme in Chicago, Bond *et al.* (1990) found that ACT subjects, in comparison to those attending a drop-in centre, spent less time in hospital, reported fewer life difficulties and were more satisfied with their care, but did not report improved quality of life generally, or differ in their housing arrangements or general level of functioning. ACT subjects remained in care during the study period to a far greater extent than control subjects.

In a random allocation study of homeless persons referred from jail, Solomon and Draine (1995a) found no differences between an assertive community treatment group, a forensic community management group or standard care on either quality of life, time spent in hospital, social adjustment, housing, subsequent arrests or substance abuse.

Non-controlled studies of ACT

In a small cross-sectional study using the OQLQ, 25 ACT patients and 17 from a comparison group were interviewed 2–3 months after discharge (Bigelow *et al.*, 1991). ACT patients reported significant improvements in the following areas: physical condition of home, structure and support of the home, total satisfaction with home, adequacy of medication, meaningful use of time, psychological distress, well-being and interpersonal relations. Bond *et al.* (1991) used a quasi-experimental design to compare ACT with an educational support reference group and a standard case management group. They found no difference between the groups on outcome measures with the exception of less substance abuse in the educational support reference group. McGrew *et al.* (1995) conducted a repeated measures design study in 212 patients receiving ACT. Quality of life was assessed using a 31-item client self-report Life Satisfaction Checklist (O'Connor-Griffin, 1990). Quality of life had improved by 6 months and showed further improvement over 18 months. Associated findings included decreased time spent in hospital and increased social adjustment ratings. Lafave *et al.* (1996) compared ACT with a hospital-based rehabilitation programme in a randomized study ($N = 110$). No baseline measures were carried out and there was considerable attrition from the study, 52 patients completing the QLI at 12 months. Those in the ACT programme scored higher on every domain of life satisfaction except health, although the differences between groups were not significant. ACT patients scored significantly higher on objective ratings in the living situation domain. In a carefully designed study, Taylor *et al.* (1998) evaluated quality of life with the QLI in comparing an intensive ACT-type service with a standard care service. This study was designed principally to determine whether randomized control trials of assertive community treatment, which generally favoured the experimental group, would sustain their effectiveness in ordinary clinical practice. Quality of life measures showed relatively little change over time in either group. There was weak evidence for an improvement in life satisfaction ratings in the living situation domain of the intensive care sector. Objective indicators of quality of life were rated low and also showed little change over time. There was a suggestion of increased social activity in the intensive sector. Hospital admissions were significantly reduced in the intensive sector and may have accounted for the improvement in satisfaction ratings in the living domain. The generally weak findings in favour of the intensive sector in this study, in such areas as social networks, carer burden, disabilities and symptoms, suggest that the outcomes frequently reported by controlled trials are less pronounced in routine clinical practice.

Controlled studies of ICM

Franklin *et al.* (1987) used the QLI to assess a programme of intensive case management (ICM) in a large study ($N = 417$) in Houston, Texas. Findings from this study were somewhat compromised by a high attrition rate. No differences were found in quality of life outcome between the case management and standard care groups. Interestingly, in this study the ICM subjects spent more time in hospital than controls.

Lehman *et al.* (1993), in a small controlled study in Baltimore, found no differences between intensive case management and standard case management groups on any outcome measures, including quality of life. This study underlines one of the problems in this series of community care studies, the small sample sizes which sometimes apply and which result in greater difficulties in finding significant differences between groups.

The problems inherent in small sample size also apply to the Swedish study of intensive case management of Aberg-Wistedt *et al.* (1995), who used the Quality of Life Self-Assessment Inventory (Skantze *et al.*, 1992). In this study, the authors reported non-significant improvements within the ICM group in quality of life, size of social network and burden of care for relatives.

In a randomized trial of social services supplied case management for long-term mental disorders, Marshall *et al.* (1995b) used the QLI to assess outcome among 80 subjects. Both experimental and control groups showed significant improvements in social behaviour (REHAB scale, Baker and Hall, 1983), and social integration (Social Integration Questionnaire, Segal and Aviram, 1977) over 14 months, but only deviant behaviour ratings favoured the case management group significantly. Neither group showed significant gains in quality of life measures or on other measures of need, quality of accommodation, employment status, social behaviour or psychopathology. The authors noted the similarities in service provision described in this study to that reported by Franklin and colleagues (1987) and noted also that that study did not favour ICM. They comment that their results challenge the orthodoxy that case management is effective.

In a small random allocation study, limited by high attrition rates and a short follow-up period, Modcrin *et al.*(1988) reported equal or better quality of life ratings for ICM over standard care patients. Other findings did not favour clear differences between the two groups.

In a random allocation study ($N = 96$) comparing two types of intensive case management, Solomon and Draine (1995b), using the OQLQ found no differences between groups on any outcome measure, including quality of life, hospitalization rates, symptoms or social adjustment.

Non-controlled studies of ICM

In a small study ($N = 30$), Cutler *et al.* (1987) examined three groups of subjects: intensive case management, standard case management and use of a social centre, and no case management. They found no differences between the groups on quality of life or other outcomes, with the exception of higher hospitalization rates for the no case management group. Bigelow and Young (1991) used the OQLQ in an outcome comparison study to compare 21 subjects receiving standard case management with 21 subjects receiving no case management. Quality of life outcome favoured the case management group, especially in the areas of well-being, social support and meaningful use of time. This finding was associated with superior housing, less time spent in hospital and lower symptoms scores for the case management group. Surles *et al.* (1992), in a pre- post-test design on 170 subjects with no comparison group found broadly positive results across a range of measures including quality of life. Lehman *et al.* (1994) assessed the efficiency of a programme developed by the Robert Wood Johnson Foundation and the US Department of Housing and Urban Development. The study was quasi-experimental in design and examined 302 subjects receiving integrated case management and 359 receiving non-integrated case management. The goal of the study was to assess whether integrated case management, following a restructuring of the service environment, which ensured continuity of care to patients, would improve functioning level and quality of life, compared with subjects receiving non-integrated standard case management. No quality of life gains were evident for the integrated case management group, perhaps reflecting the absence of any single intensive intervention that might impact sufficiently on quality of life. In a quasi-experimental design Felton *et al.* (1995) ($N = 170$) compared three groups receiving ICM, one of which was augmented with three consumer peer specialists, and another of which was augmented with three para-professionals with no previous psychiatric experience, either as patients or carers. The authors, using the QLI, found that the group featuring consumer peer specialists showed improved quality of life ratings. Subjects reported greater satisfaction with their living situation and finances and reported fewer life problems. Other outcome measures, including time in hospital or symptom levels, did not favour any one group. Jerrell and Ridgley (1995), using the life satisfaction component of the Community Adjustment Form, completed a study of quasi-experimental design comparing standard case management with pre-Alcoholic Anonymous groups and social skills training groups. Outcome measures favoured the standard case management group on quality of life but without clear differences on other outcome measures. In a study of quasi-experimental design for dually-diagnosed homeless adults, Drake *et al.* (1997) compared intensive case management for 158 patients with standard case management received by 59. Quality of life was measured using the QLI. The integrated treatment group had more days in stable housing, made more progress towards recovery from substance abuse and showed greater improvement of alcohol use disorders than the standard treatment group. Secondary outcomes such as psychiatric symptoms, functional status or quality of life also improved in both groups, but without significant group differences. Clients in both groups showed improvement in the following objective quality of life areas: finances, living skills and family contacts; and in the following life satisfaction areas: general life, housing, family relations, leisure and finances. The intensive treatment group showed a trend towards greater satisfaction with social relations and amount of social contact but the results were not significant following Bonferroni correction.

Findings from the above studies

1. It can be seen from the above studies that quality of life measures are being used with increasing regularity in mental health services research into assertive community treatment/intensive case management programmes. The ideal situation, in which a well-validated instrument is used in a controlled study, remains a relatively infrequent exercise. Fourteen of the studies of ACT or ICM in this review were of randomized control design, although sample sizes were small in some. A case has been made for research of quasi-experimental, naturalistic design to assess 'real world' effectiveness of ACT or ICM programmes, especially since earlier controlled efficacy studies have demonstrated the feasibility of these programmes. Whatever the merits of this argument generally, randomized studies of controlled design are to be preferred from the point of view of further understanding and developing quality of life tools. Quality of life instrumentation is a complex task and mental health service evaluation equally so; it makes sense, therefore, to hold as many factors constant as possible.
2. The most frequently used instrument in these studies is the QLI. Overall, however, only a minority of studies used well-validated instruments. Many used self-developed measures. Most studies would fail the requirement set by Gill and Feinstein (1994) that a theoretical justification of choice of instrument be made. A slightly jaundiced impression of some of the instruments would note an uncritical extension of 'satisfaction with service' type questions to various life domains, in the absence of sufficient consideration to structure or context.

3.   Nevertheless, the studies as a whole support the potential usefulness of quality of life outcome measurement in health services research. A review of ACT studies in 1990 (Olfson, 1990) concluded that, apart from the original programme in Madison, Wisconsin, quality of life was not shown to be improved by the use of intensive treatment services. The number of studies with a positive quality of life outcome reviewed in this chapter suggests that Olfson's negative conclusion may no longer be applicable. Of the 25 studies that assessed quality of life in this review, nine reported improvement. This suggests that quality of life measurement may have a valid role in assessing the outcome of community care programmes.

4.   Are quality of life measures sufficiently sensitive to warrant a place within outcome studies?. An interesting example of the potential role of quality of life as an outcome measure is contained in a recent paper from Rosenheck et al. (1998) who used the Quality of Life Scale (Heinrichs et al., 1984) to assess whether the use of a psychosocial treatment programme mediates the clinical effectiveness of clozapine. Clozapine facilitated participation in psychosocial treatment, and this enhanced participation was associated with improved quality of life and symptom outcomes one year later. The Quality of Life Scale functioned as a useful indicator of proximal outcome in this study which found that improvement in quality of life relative to standard medication became evident at 6 months, more than 4 months after the emergence of differential symptom improvement and 3 months after the appearance of significant differences in participation in psychosocial treatment. Browne et al. (1996) also reported significant improvement on Quality of Life Scale ratings following a psychosocial and educative rehabilitation programme, and Atkinson et al. (1996) too reported significant improvement following a group education programme. It is not possible to draw firm conclusions from the series of studies in this review because a variety of instruments, some non-validated, have been used. However, of the 16 studies that reported both quality of life and social adjustment outcomes (two further studies were excluded because of mixed results), eight reported improved quality of life as against four reporting improved social adjustment. Thus, these studies suggest that quality of life may be as sensitive as, or more sensitive than, social adjustment as an outcome indicator. Further instrument development for use in these types of trials may well enhance sensitivity, particularly if attention is directed towards increasing measurement sensitivity to change over time, as in the suggested use of transition scoring (Ziebland, 1994).

5.   Most of the standard instruments that have been used to assess quality of life in these studies were originally developed within a context of rehabilitation or community aftercare programmes and they therefore

reflect social rather than clinical determinants of quality of life. Thus, in the first group of studies described in this chapter, change in quality of life status was likely to be prominently reflected in the living situation domain. It is of interest, therefore, that in a recent review of ACT/ICM studies, Mueser *et al.* (1998) noted that improvement in quality of life, in addition to being associated with living situation, was also associated with reduction in symptoms or time in hospital. Conversely, of the studies that failed to register any improvement in quality of life, two-thirds also failed to register reductions in either symptoms or time spent in hospital. These associations may therefore reflect an enduring clinical dimension to the determination of quality of life outcome in these studies. Kaiser *et al.* (1997), in their evaluation of schizophrenic patients, noted that clinical status contributed to about 30% of quality of life variance. This prompts the question whether the dominance of social over clinical determinants of quality of life, as pertains in most current quality of life instruments, ought to be maintained. Instead of efforts towards progressive exclusion of psychopathological factors (Katschnig, 1997), then, at the risk of some measurement redundancy, it may be that quality of life measurement should reflect both clinical and social influences, in a holistic fashion.

General conclusion

Quality of life measurement has been seen to play an increasing role in the evaluation of health services. Many of the standard instruments were developed with a view to the evaluation of broad socially-based influences. Despite this, and despite the inclusion of self-developed scales in a number of studies, quality of life measurement emerges as a reasonably sensitive outcome indicator. Further instrument development to increase sensitivity to the evaluation of changes over time may enhance the relevance of quality of life measurement in this area of research.

4

How to use quality of life measures in individual care

JOSEPH P.J. OLIVER

Introduction

The addition of the concept of quality of life to our ideas about health and health services is proving to be one of the most important advances in our thinking to have occurred during the past decade. It is helping us to move from a much narrower, symptom-centred view of individuals with mental health problems towards a more holistic view acknowledging the myriad of human predicaments in which they find themselves entangled. This leads us inevitably towards a consideration of the wider ramifications of our treatments, the implications of various models of viewing health and what our expectations might be of services and the professionals employed to provide them, taking into account the overall well-being of our patients.

One important challenge for quality of life scales is for them to become integrated into the usual workings of mental health services. However, observing the organization and finance of UK mental health services, as recently as 1994, the Audit Commission (1994) commented on the 'almost complete absence of information concerning outcomes' and the need to promote outcomes which concentrate on measuring 'quality' dimensions of users' concerns. Recently, this observation has been reconfirmed in the UK Department of Health initiative to develop high performance indicators. At commencement, the exercise only proposed two outcome measures for mental health: the suicide rate in the general population and the rate of psychiatric readmissions. It noted the need for outcomes measures as an area for development and the need for user based quality of life indicators specifically (National Health Service Executive, 1998).

In their review, Fitzpatrick et al. (1992) observe that, in reality, clinicians remain unconvinced of the ultimate value of quality of life assessments, despite the fact that in many other areas of health care, quality of life assessments have been accepted. Various reasons for this scepticism appear to exist.

One potential reason cited is that some approaches to quality of life appear too philosophical for clinicians. The inclusion of more general notions such as life satisfaction or living standards are cited by Fitzpatrick *et al.* (1992) as two examples which are generally excluded from clinical assessment in favour of more limited measures of health related quality of life. These might include only health status and/or functional ability. Also, many clinicians seem unswayed by the presence of considerable evidence that clinical judgements differ markedly from those made by patients of themselves. Apparently, according to Spitzer *et al.* (1981), the presence of these systematic differences does not lead clinicians to alter their views by taking on board new information. Rather, they lead clinicians to mistrust the rating measures. Ignoring the information, thus, in turn reinforces in clinicians' minds its lack of relevancy.

Importantly, the form of feedback from measures is identified as being a crucial variable in acceptance. Quality of life information may be ignored because it is 'not fed back to clinicians in the most useful format or at the right time' (Fitzpatrick *et al.*, 1992). In considering the nature of this dilemma, this chapter will focus on the matter of length as a principal hurdle to be overcome in having quality of life measures accepted into routine clinical practice. An innovation in quality of life assessment concerning the form of feedback will be discussed as a potential means of overcoming clinical resistance.

A comparison of selected measures

Despite the mass of literature existing about quality of life, relatively little research has been undertaken on the matter of length of measures and there are few conclusive facts around which to build a theory. Hence, this chapter is exploratory and much of what is written is necessarily speculative. What is certain is that researchers are now confronted with a spectrum of scales, checklists, structured and semi-structured interviews which, according to one's definition, can be classified reasonably as quality of life scales. Not surprisingly, the categorization of quality of life measures has become a very ambitious task. There are only a few useful articles that systematically and critically evaluate the range of quality of life measures available. An examination of the existing literature via a keyword search of PsychLIT (Psychological Abstracts) and Medline (Index Medicus) CD-ROM databases for the past 10 years exposed only a handful of useful references (e.g. Rosser *et al.*, 1992; Fitzpatrick *et al.*, 1992; Bowling, 1995; Lehman, 1996; Barry and Zissi, 1997). Two of these, Bowling, 1995 and Lehman, 1996, are well constructed general reviews of the field which touch on the matter of length of measure and form the basis of much of what is discussed below.

Table I. Mental health quality of life instruments: psychiatric rating scales.

Title	Author(s)	Type of instrument	No. of items	No. of domains	Completion time
Brief Psychiatric Rating Scale (BPRS)	Overall and Gorham, 1962	Symptom checklist: Clinician	18 items		
Symptom Checklist (SCL-90)	Parloff et al., 1954	Symptom checklist: Self-report	90 items	9 sub-scales	20 min
Brief Symptom Inventory (BSI)	Derogatis, 1993	Symptom checklist: Self-report	53 items	9 sub-scales	8–10 min
Symptom Rating Test	Kellner and Sheffield, 1973	Symptom checklist: Clinician	37 items	4 sub-scales	
Rand Depression Screener	Burnham et al., 1988	Depression checklist	8 items	1	10 min
General Health Questionnaire (GHQ)	Goldberg, 1972	Psychiatric screening: Self-report	Q60, 30, 28 and 12 items	4 sub-scales	
Beck Depression Inventory (BDI)	Beck et al., 1961	Depression checklist: Self or interviewer	21 items	1	10–15 min
Profile of Mood States (POMs)	McNair et al., 1971	Mood scale	65 items	6 aspects of mood	

Bowling (1995) reviews the full range of quality of life measures being employed in health. She included not only those measures which may genuinely be regarded as 'true' quality of life measures (i.e. quality of life measurement was their stated purpose and their contents cover an appropriate range of issues). She also reviews those measures that have come to be regarded as quality of life measures though they fall outside of this definition (e.g. 'domain specific' or 'health related' quality of life measures). Drawing on information taken principally from her very informative chapter on quality of life measures of 'psychiatric condition and psychological morbidity', the Tables 1–4 have been constructed. Each table summarizes a sample of instruments according to title, author(s), and type of scale. In addition length is described according to number of items contained in the measure, the number of domains covered and the completion time. As this chapter is based on an exploration of secondary sources, the parameters examined are limited by what the original reviewers chose to include in their

Table 2. Mental health quality of life instruments: complex quality of life interviews.

Title	Author(s)	Type of instrument	No. of items	No. of domains	Completion time
Quality of Life Scale	Heinrichs et al., 1984	Symptoms and functioning: Trained clinician	21 items	4	45 min
Quality of Life Interview (QLI)	Lehman, 1988	Structured interview: Interviewer	200 items	10	45 min
Lancashire Quality of Life Interview (LQOLP)	Oliver, 1991a	Structured interview: Interviewer	108 items	11	35 min
SmithKline Beecham Quality of Life (SBQOL)	Dunbar et al., 1992	Structured interview: Self-report	78 items (?)	23	
Oregon Quality of Life Interview	Bigelow et al., 1990	Semi-structured and self-report interview	263 items	14 scales	40–40 min
Index of Health-Related Quality of Life	Rosser et al., 1992	Disability, emotional distress and physical discomfort interview	107 descriptors and 225 descriptor levels between them	3 domains	
Quality of Life Index for Mental Health (QLI-MH)	Becker et al., 1993	Self-report and interviewer questionnaire	160+ items	15+ domains	10–30 min
General Well-Being Scale (GWBS)	Dupuy, 1973	Positive and negative affect: Self-report	22 items	2 domains	12 min

descriptions of instruments and relies on their accuracy. Only scales where sufficient relevant information was readily accessible have been reported on here. The purpose of this compilation is not an exhaustive cataloguing of measures but rather to provide a comparative view of a range of what exists and to explore what useful observations might be drawn from looking at a selection of their main parameters.

Table 1 summarizes eight conventional psychiatric rating scales currently being used as quality of life instruments. Under the heading of 'Complex quality of life Interviews', Table 2 summarizes information concerning eight instruments, which might be considered 'true' quality of life instruments in the sense that each was designed specifically for that task and is multidimensional. Table 3 lists details of four instruments designed to measure role functioning and adjustment, also being employed as quality of life measures. Table 4 lists seven instruments that measure quality of life in non-psychiatric conditions such as asthma, cancer and epilepsy.

Table 3. Mental health quality of life instruments: role functioning and related instruments

Title	Author(s)	Type of instrument	No. of items	No. of domains	Completion time
Social Dysfunction Rating Scale	Linn et al., 1969	Functional rating scale: Trained clinician	21 items	3 domains: self, interpersonal relations and dissatisfaction in social situations	
Structured and Scaled Interview to Assess Maladjustment (SSIAM)	Gurland et al., 1972	Social maladjustment: Trained interviewer	60 items	8 domains	30–45 min
Social Adjustment Scale-II (SAS-II) and Self-Report Version	Paykel et al., 1971	Functional measure of interpersonal relationships: Interviewer and self-report versions	54 items	6 domains: work/school (18); leisure (11); family (7); marital (9); parent (4); family member (4)	Interviewer version: 60 min; Self administered version: 10 min
Psychosocial Adjustment to Illness Scale (PAIS)	Morrow et al., 1978	Psychological or social adjustment to illness: Interviewer and self-report versions	46 items	7 domains	30 min (both versions)

Table 5 is drawn from the work of Lehman, (1996) who reviewed 10 'humanistic' quality of life measures. This was a carefully selected set of mental health quality of life measures that met predetermined criteria including focusing on the assessment of subjective well-being and the availability of sufficient information describing them. In Lehman's selection, all measures took the form of structured, semi-structured interviews or checklists – half took 45 min to administer; 2/10 took longer. One was very brief, taking only 10 min to complete. The number of questions contained in each varied accordingly: 140 items/45 min, 93 items/60 min, 15 items/10 min, 263 or 146 items/45 min, 143 items/45 min, 21 items/45 min, 46 items/30 min, 151 items/unknown; 100 items/55 min. Lehman's analysis identified three measures as being of particular utility for work with the severely mentally ill: The Quality of Life Interview (143 items/45 min); the Oregon Quality of Life Interview (93 items/60 min) and the Lancashire Quality of life Profile (100 items/35–55 min).

Table 4. Non-psychiatric conditions: quality of life instruments.

Title	Author(s)	Type of instrument	No. of items	No. of domains	Completion time
Living with Asthma Questionnaire	Hyland et al., 1991	Quality of Life for Asthma: Interviewer or Self-report	68 items	12 domains: e.g. social, leisure, sport, sleep, attitudes, medications	15–20 min
Washington Psychosocial Inventory	Dodrill 1978	Quality of Life for Epilepsy: Self-report	132 items	8 domains: e.g. overall functioning: adjustment	15–20 min
Epilepsy Surgery Inventory (ESI-55)	Vickrey et al., 1992	Quality of life for epilepsy: Self-report	55 items	11 health domains	15 min
Hornquist Quality of Life Status and Change Scale	Hornquist et al., 1993	Quality of life for rheumatoid arthritis: Self-report	34 items	6 domains: somatic, psychological, social, behavioural, structural, material	
European Organization for Research on Treatment of Cancer (EORTC-30)	Aaronson, 1993	Quality of life for cancer: Self-report	30 core items + 13 disease specific items	9 domains: 5 functional: 3 symptom; 1 global well-being	10 min
Rotterdam Symptom Checklist	de Haes et al., 1990	Quality of life for cancer: Self-report	38 items	4 domains	5–10 min
Quality of Life Index	Ferrans and Powers, 1985	Quality of life for cancer: Self-report	64 items	4 domains: health, socio-economic, psychological, family	

The quality of life measures listed above (Tables 1–5) cover a wide variety of types of instrument. It would seem that those interviews applying to the mentally ill tend to be longer and are more likely to have an interview format. Self-report is visibly less popular with mental health measures than with non-psychiatric ones. For mental health ratings, the number of questions asked typically exceeds 50 and it is not uncommon to find an instrument with more than 100 items. The number and types of domains vary considerably with all but two measuring between four and 15 domains. Times taken in interview range from 10 min to 1 hour. Typically, mental health ratings appear to take longer than non-psychiatric ones to complete.

The World Health Organization Quality of Life Assessment (WHOQOL) has not been included above only because of its developmental nature. On

Table 5. Ten 'humanistic' quality of life instruments.

Title	Author(s)	No. of items	No. of domains	Completion time
Standardized Social Schedule	Clare and Cairns, 1978	48	6	45 min
Community Adjustment Form	Stein and Test, 1980	140	12	45 min
Quality of Life Checklist	Malm et al., 1981	93	11	60 min
Satisfaction with Life Domains Scale	Baker and Intagliata, 1982	15	15	10 min
Oregon Quality of Life Scale	Bigelow et al., 1991	146	14	45 min
Lehman Quality of Life Interview	Lehman, 1988	143	8	45 min
Quality of Life Scale	Heinrichs et al., 1984	21	21	45 min
Client Quality of Life Interview	Mulkern et al., 1986	65	8	30 min
Well-Being Project Client Interview	Campbell, et al., 1989	151, 76 and 77	60	Not known
Lancashire Quality of Life Interview	Oliver, 1991a	100	11	35–50 min

the basis of available information, it will be composed of 100 items, spanning six domains and 24 facet scores. Time required for the interview is not known (WHOQOL Group, 1995).

How brief is 'brief'? The instance of the single-item scale

Thus far, various forms of instrumentation have been largely excluded from our considerations. Single-item scales are not included and are not generally recommended whereas multi-item scales have been indicated to be superior in various respects. Single-item scales are thought to be popular because they are brief and easy to administer and analyse. It is doubtful whether single questions can effectively tap and measure a given domain. It is also difficult to fully assess their reliability (e.g. they cannot be split for multiple forms or split-half reliability testing) (Bowling, 1995,). Several investigators have shown how single-item measures are more likely to fall short of the minimum level of precision needed for testing hypotheses because of their coarseness (Bowling, 1995). Some questionnaires such as the Hornquist Quality of Life

Status and Change Scale are said to be insensitive, probably due to their brevity (i.e. most scales have as few as one or at most three questions). As mentioned above (Fitzpatrick *et al.*, 1992), there is an established consensus that quality of life is a multidimensional construct requiring multidimensional measures, and short measures have tended to violate this principle by being overly simple.

In an illustrative report, Spitzer *et al.* (1981) discuss the motivations of clinicians for wanting to develop short questionnaires. Like other clinicians, those authors had found many reasons to be displeased with the various quality of life and health status instruments that they encountered. In respect of the length and function of the measures that they found, they reported that the scales that they were presented with for assessing global health or quality of life were usually lengthy, required specially trained research personnel to administer, code and store the information, and represented an expensive exercise. They concluded that these had limited use out of the research setting because physicians find them too long or complicated for routine, periodic assessment of patients (Spitzer *et al.*, 1981). They specifically cite the Sickness Impact Profile (Bergner *et al.*, 1976) which they reported (apparently unhappily) as containing '312 items in 14 categories' (Spitzer *et al.*, 1981).

In creating the Multiscale (10 questions), the QL-Index (five questions) and the QL-Uniscale (one question) the same authors aimed to test three measures, as well as meeting the various scientific exigencies of reliability and validity. They demanded that, first and foremost, a measure 'should be simple, which means it should be short, easy to understand, to remember, to administer and to record' (Spitzer *et al.*, 1981). This they accomplished. For example, the QL-Index was found to have an average completion time of one minute. However, they concluded that short was not found ultimately to be best. In their study, 'the simplest rating scale, the Uniscale was least preferred' (Spitzer *et al.*, 1981). While their measures did satisfy practitioners (i.e. they accurately depicted practitioners' views of patients' life quality), they were persistently inaccurate (i.e. systematically underestimated patient responses) and were of limited use on their own. They concluded that their efforts did not 'discriminate adequately among well people. It would seem that there are no shortcuts to the long, comprehensive questionnaires such as the Sickness Impact Profile (SIP) to assess the physical, social and emotional functions of people living freely in the community' (Spitzer *et al.*, 1981).

Likewise, many extremely lengthy batteries of tests exist (Bowling, 1991; 1995). Some of these have included up to 10 different questionnaires. Data were not available to describe their length, i.e. number of items and time required for application. Nevertheless, there is little doubt that the routine employment in mental health services of such extremely lengthy batteries is unlikely. It is likely that managers would resist their usage on grounds of economy and because of apprehension that the service purposes of the organization might become skewed by the research enterprise. As these would be impractical to recommend for routine clinical practice, they have not been considered above.

Self-report versus interviewer administered measurements

One important predictor of resistance to worker usage is the amount of professional time being taken to administer a measure. In general, the measure requiring the minimum of direct staff input is, of course, the self-report measure. Here the only clinicians' time required may be to hand the questionnaire to the patient, if that. There is a temptation to view this as the least expensive and least 'troublesome' option.

However, at this time self-report questionnaires should be regarded as less applicable to people with severe mental illnesses. The severely mentally ill frequently suffer from a defect state, and negative symptoms such as apathy and withdrawal make completion of questionnaires more difficult. Various aspects of thought disorder can diminish the ability of the subject to concentrate. Auditory hallucinations are intrusive and may affect reliability. People with affective disorder either can be too easily distracted to concentrate or too withdrawn to complete the task on their own (Bowling, 1995). Overall, 'significant numbers of these patients have problems with task perseverance and comprehension. Therefore, pencil and paper questionnaires are ill-advised' (Lehman, 1996).

Another important matter rests in the inclusion or exclusion of clinical measures supplementary to quality of life in the same interview. It has been established that mental state can affect quality of life scores (Lehman, 1983b). It is, therefore, advised that the administration of quality of life scales with the severely mentally ill be accompanied by some, even if minimal, assessment of mental state, especially mood. This inclusion necessarily increases both the total number of domains examined, the total number of questions posed, as well as the interview time required. In addition, there may be a degree of subject reactivity to quality of life interviewing (Oliver *et al.*, 1996; Lehman, 1996). This probably results from the exercise of considering one's life in itself. Potential lowering of mood must be identified and dealt with where appropriate as this is not simply of scientific interest but may be clinically relevant, translating into exacerbated symptoms. A clinically trained professional (e.g. one of the specialist members of a multi-disciplinary mental health team) is best equipped for this task and a psychiatric interview is the appropriate context.

Self-administered quality of life scales, such as the Quality of Life Index for Mental Health (QLI-MH) by Becker *et al.* (1993), have tried to address some of these problems directly during construction. However, reflecting the concerns enumerated above, their general acceptance has yet to be witnessed. For example, in a subsequent paper (Sanifort *et al.*, 1996), the authors of the QLI-MH have reported the modest to nil associations achieved during a structured trial between this self-report scale and an independent measure.

In discussing the matter of questionnaire format, Bowling (1995) considers the virtues of self-report and interviewer administered questionnaires. She makes the following excellent points relevant to the length of interviews: 'The method of choice will often be determined by practical considerations, such as the financial resources available for the research and the condition of the patient, as well as the length of the instrument. Methodological considerations may pose a paradox for the researcher. Concise, self-report scales are cheaper to administer and analyse, they can be sent by post or given to respondents to complete themselves in the presence of an interviewer, and they are less taxing for respondents. However, they may be insufficiently sensitive and informative to answer the research question. Short questionnaires inevitably lose sensitivity, and postal questionnaires have to be short and simple. Long interview questionnaires or longer batteries of self-report scales may sometimes be preferable, but they are expensive to administer and analyse, and longer batteries of self-report scales usually require an interviewer to administer them, or to at least explain their instructions. Interviewer-administered questionnaires may also include some self-report scales to be given to respondents to complete during the interview. These usually result in better quality data because ambiguities can be explained, assistance can be given where necessary (e.g. with reading), in-depth information can be collected and the good rapport between the interviewer and the interviewee usually leads to a better overall item response rate' (Bowling, 1995).

Domains and items: what is the correct balance?

The classic work of Andrews and Withey (1976) considered the measurement of social indicators – a type of life quality measure. They searched for 'a limited yet comprehensive set of coherent and significant indicators, which can be monitored over time, and which can be disaggregated to the level of the relevant social unit'. Andrews and Withey have provided future investigators with useful guidelines for the production of quality of life scales as they relate to both social and health phenomena. They maintained that a set of measures 'should be "limited" so they can be understandable and not overly detailed, lengthy, or complex. The indicators should be "comprehensive" so that a substantial quota of the salient or critical aspects of society are included. They should be "coherent" in that it would be helpful to our understanding if they hung together in some form that would eventually lead to a model or theory about how society operates. Any set of indicators would be "significant" if they fulfilled the foregoing demands but there is a further implication that they should be of "direct normative interest", which implies that they should relate to aspects of society that interest or concern us'.

It is noteworthy that, like other investigators of the time (e.g. Campbell *et al.*, 1976), Andrews and Withey (1976) identified the need to focus life quality investigation on areas of real human concern. They defined life domains as those sorts of concerns relative to 'places, things, activities, people and roles'. In constructing measures of these domains, they demonstrated the need to consider both objective indicators, i.e. judgements made by others about our social or health state as well as subjective indicators, i.e. our own judgements about these external circumstances. Both types of life quality indicators are necessary and desirable while it is individuals' perceptions 'of their own well-being, or lack of well-being, that ultimately define the quality of their lives'. Though writers come from different professional orientations and nationalities, the contributors have supported this view through this book.

The number of domains

There is little doubt that the effective type and number of domains will vary from one quality of life measure to another. Employing a multiple regression technique, Andrews and Withey (1976) looked closely at the number of predictors required to reliably identify 'perceived quality of life' (a series of subjective individual perceptions about a range of human concerns). They conclude that from an original set of 30 life concerns drawn from and tested on large populations, 'only a certain heterogeneous nine are really needed for maximal predictions of feeling about life-as-a-whole, and close-to-maximal levels can be obtained with just six. Even using as few as four or five can be almost as effective. If a dozen predictors are used, there is sufficient overlap among them that the removal of one does not produce a marked decrement in explanatory power'. However, maximizing the amount of explained variance with the minimum number of variables is only one element in the solution of establishing a valid means of assessing such a wide concept as quality of life. They warn future would-be investigators that 'we do not propose that assessment of only these few particular concerns would in any way constitute an adequate monitoring effort from a social indicators perspective. Ability to account for differences in feeling about life-as-a-whole is certainly not the only requirement of a set of indicators' (Andrews and Withey, 1976).

Three results crucial to our considerations emerge from the work of Andrews and Withey:

1. That any set of nine concerns, sometimes referred to as life domains, which cover the breadth of likely concerns of a population (i.e. are heterogeneous) are likely to produce an acceptable account of subjective feelings about life as a whole,
2. That heterogeneous sets of concerns are of more predictive value in respect to appraisals of general well-being than are homogeneous ones (by an average of 40%),
3. That the predictive power of a given homogeneous set of concerns depends on the particular concept area that it addresses, for instance, concerns about one's neighbourhood or locality, though important, may prove to be only a fraction as predictive of general-well-being as feelings about one's 'self'; also, the actual individual items used to measure concerns, though important, are secondary in importance to the particular conceptual area that they address.

These findings help to illuminate the utility of the quality of life scales listed in Tables 1–5 above. Some critical characteristics are the focus on the production of a multidimensional overview; addressing a heterogeneous range of concerns in preference to a homogeneous one, a tendency to cover no fewer than six but more frequently nine domains, and containing or being designed to be used alongside mood measures.

Form follows function

Considering the above, the content of any clinical rating scale, be it a diagnostic measure, a health status measure or a quality of life measure, may be determined by many factors. However, the guiding principle for the construction and selection of instruments appropriate for routine organizational and clinical use within modern human service organizations is clearer, i.e. form must follow function (supported by Lehman, 1996). This dictum decrees that while the structure and content of a measure may vary, it must follow on from the use for which it is intended. This should seem apparent but in the case of quality of life measures it is not. There are now a large number of potential measures from which to choose. What seems baffling is not that measures differ but rather the dilemma of trying to choose the most appropriate measure for the given set of circumstances. For this task, no essential research exists currently. Hence, while this chapter can only endorse a rather pragmatic approach to the matter, in doing so one has the consolation that choosing because of function does guarantee that whatever measure is used, it is relevant or 'fit for purpose'.

It must be acknowledged that alternative selection principles exist. One alternative approach which might prove especially attractive to administrators, and which is in keeping with many of the concerns relating to the economies of information gathering with this client group, might be called *the resource allocation approach*. According to this model, form is determined by cost and priority. The principal method for employing this model might be to identify available resources, to determine levels of need, to determine priorities, and to cost alternatives. The form of a quality of life measure would be determined by adhering to the most economical criteria. In reality, many considerations need to be taken into account in instrument design.

The purposes to which psychiatric rating scales in general and quality of life scales in particular may be put

Researchers may think of psychiatric rating scales, particularly quantitative ones, as having specific uses such as interview guides, communication, record of treatment progress and research (Research and Education Association, 1981). Interview guides are regarded as important to clinicians. A list of items covering a range of symptoms or relevant questions concerning a patient's affect, thoughts, perceptions or behaviour helps to ensure consistent, thorough and complete psychiatric examinations. It is often critical not to overlook vital information, particularly in such tasks as assessing risks, whether or not the information being gathered is subsequently used for statistical purposes. One presumes that this may apply especially to complex cases such as those frequently encountered when dealing with patients with severe and chronic mental disorders and their families. Communication can be enhanced and improved by ensuring that all those passing information share definitions and understandings. Unlike purely narrative descriptions, quantitative reports and checklists of symptoms are less likely to be misinterpreted. In multidisciplinary work, when professionals emanate from different cultural and theoretical backgrounds, misunderstanding is easy and, as in the too frequent and tragic cases seen in community care, can have disastrous results. It is vital to record information in an agreed format, as aid to future clarification. This is also important where records or information gained from them is being passed along, accompanying a patient through a system. This would include when patients are being first referred, later discharged from care, or transferred. The task of maintaining a record of treatment progress is facilitated by the availability of a valid set of rating scales that correspond to the particular condition. Numerical or graphical presentations of change, either of progress or deterioration in symptoms or other aspects of the patient's disorder, are useful for following observable trends in the course of change. Finally, useful research relies on objective data, 'data that can be manipulated statistically, data that have sufficient dependability (reliability), data obtained in such a way that other researchers can repeat the study in an attempt to confirm or challenge the original findings. Modern research designs demand information in numerical form, derived from the same instrument or instruments, and gathered in a uniform or reproducible manner. Well constructed rating scales, as other psychometric devices when properly used, meet most of the requirements of today's experimental and statistical procedures' (Research and Education Association, 1981).

Quality of life measures, like psychiatric rating scales in general, may be put to the above uses. Nevertheless, they have a much wider variety of established uses as well as some potential uses that have not been fully described. Fitzpatrick *et al.* (1992) explored the different ways in which quality of life measures can be used within health care, particularly attending to the fact that a given instrument or measurement technique may prove valid and reliable for one task or setting but not for another. The six useful applications as identified by Fitzpatrick *et al.* (1992) are:

1. Screening and monitoring for psychosocial problems in individual patient care,
2. Population surveys of perceived health problems,
3. Medical audit,
4. Outcome measures in health services or evaluation research,
5. Clinical trials, and
6. Cost–utility analysis.

Our own current research in the North West of England on the Lancashire Quality of Life Profiling Project, appears to be identifying a seventh:

7. As a clinical tool for the formulation of care plans and a vehicle for engaging severely mentally ill patients in community care.

Quality of life instrument functions and criteria for selection

Without exhaustively examining each function some points are quite apparent. To date, quality of life has been used most widely in respect of population surveys, as an outcome measure for evaluative research and as a measure for clinical trials. There is a very considerable body of published work in these areas and it would be possible to examine this work by careful meta-analysis, linking particular questionnaires with particular functions. Certainly, many of the above instruments have been employed for one or more of these functions. Ultimately, for these functions one could be optimistic about determining the optimal lengths and contents of quality of life instruments on an empirical basis, i.e. that which appears to work best.

Both modern health and social care organizations are charged with the related tasks of determining need and designing service provisions accordingly. Efforts which have been made in the UK to achieve this on the basis of existing sociodemographic, morbidity, mortality, patient flow and employee activity information have proven difficult and of questionable validity. These are surrogate measures that have inevitably been found to lack the sensitivity necessary for providing a basis for planning and expenditure. Effective resource allocation requires additional information about both general populations and individual service users. Also, the increasing emphasis on employing public health models of health care delivery requires knowledge about local and national variations in health status, among patient groups. Demonstrating that inequalities which exist in health status and health care within the population emanate from differences in demographic characteristics such as gender, age, ethnicity, educational attainment and housing class enhances the case for a public health approach. Quality of life surveys might be thought of as one way of enhancing the utility of an existing information base.

The purpose of a clinical trial is to prove, in the most unambiguous fashion possible, the effectiveness of a particular intervention. This includes the potential benefits of treatment as well as the costs and potential risks to patients' health and well-being. According to Fitzpatrick et al. (1992) and Fitzpatrick (1994), it is in the area of clinical trials in which quality of life measures have received most attention. The complex nature of mental health aetiologies and treatment packages determines that single, standard outcomes such as mortality are not adequate. Here, quality of life measures 'provide invaluable evidence of the effects of interventions. Unfortunately, many trials purporting to assess impact of treatment on quality of life do not assess the construct properly or assess a single or limited aspect of what is a multidimensional construct' (Fitzpatrick et al., 1992). This may make conducting an analysis similar to that proposed above problematic. According to research cited by Fitzpatrick (1994), Guyatt et al. (1989) reviewed the employment of health status measures in clinical trials and found them employed in only 10 of 55 studies. This is beginning to be taken on board by clinical investigators and the LQOLP is currently being employed as a main outcome measure in the 30-site national UK trial SOS for the new drug, quetiapine, by Zeneca Pharmaceuticals (Clinical Trial 5077UK/001).

Certainly, there is increased pressure on the part of health services administrators to achieve an efficient service and correspondingly an increased burden on providers of clinical services to demonstrate that they are providing a value for money service. Health Related Quality of Life (HRQL) is systematically being related to cost–utility analysis (Ebrahim, 1995). Such a limited (i.e. impairment, disability, or handicap) model of quality of life is over-simplistic and far too inadequate conceptually for work with the severely mentally disordered. Because of the broad all-encompassing nature of psychiatric impairment and the lack of specificity of effect of psychiatric care, it can safely be assumed that employment of a narrow set of outcomes, such as those proposed by some HRQL advocates is never justified. For instance, Wilkinson *et al.* (1992) illustrated the limitations of the one-dimensional Quality Adjusted Life Years (QALYs).

Screening psychiatric patients would seem to be a less commonly employed use for quality of life measures but one which is clearly established. The purpose of a screening exercise in health care is to identify problems in a population that might have gone otherwise unnoticed and untreated. Early detection and early intervention are supposed to be more effective in preventing mortality and/or chronic course, by catching a condition before it progresses to a fully blown clinical case. Effective screening might lead to reduced distress, improved general health and reduced costs to the system.

Above all things, screening instruments need to be able to accurately distinguish one condition from another and to do so under conditions requiring briefer measures. They must be able to establish a diagnosis quickly and lead to scientifically reliable classifications (Bowling, 1995). The accuracy of a screening test is 'determined by its sensitivity, specificity and predictive value. Sensitivity is the proportion of individuals with a disease that a test detects. Specificity is the proportion of individuals without the disease so identified by the test. Predictive value is probably the criterion of most relevance to a health professional using a screening test in clinical practice. It is concerned with the proportion of all those predicted by the test as having a disease who prove to have the disease.' (Fitzpatrick, 1994). These measures tend to brief and quick to complete. Among others, the 18-item BPRS (Overall and Gorham, 1962), the 12-item version of the GHQ (Goldberg, 1972), the 21-item Quality of Life Scale (Heinrichs *et al.*, 1984) and, of course, the Quality of Life Uniscale (Spitzer *et al.*, 1981) are used this way. However, at the other end of the spectrum, the Quality of Life Checklist (93 items) (Malm *et al.*, 1981) also has been used for screening. Also, it must be noted that some of these measures depend upon clinical judgements rather than on subjective appraisals made by the patient. This means that they must be used very judiciously.

Medical audit is a performance management procedure for improving the quality of a service. It basically entails staff undertaking a joint systematic stock take of specific aspects of their service. The data are generally gathered by staff from staff about dimensions of patient care, as seen through their own eyes, and then analysed. There is no clear pattern for quality of life usage in medical audit but audit does not involve eliciting patient/user opinion but a focus on the quantifiable dimensions of a service, frequently activity levels of staff. A summary quality of life measure made by staff (e.g. Spitzer *et al.*, 1981) could be used as an estimate and even if wildly inadequate, should prove a useful addition to audit procedures because of the focus on patient concerns (see Audit Commission, 1994).

Our group in Manchester has been continually impressed with the favourable reaction of service users to quality of life interviewing. Within the North West of England, there is currently an active programme of development under way, the purpose of which is to make quality of life assessments part and parcel of routine clinical practice, called the Quality of Life Profiling Project.

'Profiling' is defined as the the act of constructing an outline, framework or short biographical sketch. A profile may require further details in order to represent a complete picture. 'Quality of life profiling' is a way of making a psycho–social–medical assessment of an individual's current state of well-being or health and welfare. Like any such assessment, quality of life profiling implies a brief but comprehensive interview, initiated by the clinician but requiring the full cooperation of the subject. The estimated result from profiling is intended first and foremost for clinical purposes. Profiling is not designed to be a means of rationing health care or treatment and should not be confused with other techniques that are (e.g. QALYs). One might look at profiling as a format for single case assessment and analysis.

The Lancashire Quality of Life Profile (LQOLP) is, of course, a tool for profiling and the LQOLP Analytical Software for Windows is designed to facilitate this development.

The Lancashire Quality of Life Profiling Project derives from the observation that patients who have completed the LQOLP seem especially well disposed to engaging in the development and use of a systematic care plan, an essential ingredient in successful case management. This effect does not appear to accompany all other therapeutic or care management activities. The way in which the use of quality of life interviews appears to help to engage clients in ongoing care or treatment has been reported (Oliver *et al.*, 1996) and has been observed in clinical practice during the current trials, but has not been systematically investigated. This is a genuine discovery, very cutting edge and with profound implications both for practice and research.

A second keyword search of PsychLIT and Medline (quality of life and mental) was made and from the more than 600 references identified only one relevant reference was identified. A paper by Skantze and Malm (1994) approaches the issue and seems to lend support to the observation. The authors describe the Quality of Life Self-Assessment Inventory approach (QLS-100) which appears to promote the development of working alliances between mental health service delivery staff and persons with schizophrenia or other mental illness. The QLS-100 helps devise successful treatment programmes tailored for individual patients; it describes specific needs and demonstrates the array of skills required for personal effectiveness and specific patient aspirations in each particular case. In the paper, case examples of QLS-100 assessment of two patients are presented. Working alliances can be successfully maintained when regularly performed QLS-100 assessments are taken into account together with the need to check the effectiveness of services, to record changes in needs, and to revise plans in collaboration with the patient and her or his family network (PsychLIT Copyright 1994, American Psychological Association).

In their important recent publication, the Royal Pharmaceutical Society of Great Britain (1997) reviewed the area of compliance with treatment. They have determined that for all chronic conditions considered together, only approximately 50% of patients continue to take their medications as prescribed. This low success rate at keeping patients in continuing therapy has the obvious effects of reducing treatment impact and increasing costs spectacularly. A review of research in respect of medical specialities (e.g. antihypertensive therapy) indicates that, although the degrees may vary according to specific conditions, hundreds of thousands of deaths occur and many hundreds of millions of pounds of money may be wasted as a result of treatment non-compliance. This regular failure to achieve the benefits of health treatments applies equally to severely mentally ill people with chronic illnesses.

To combat this terrible waste of health resources and startling health loss to patients, the Royal Pharmaceutical Society (1997) conclude that a variety of steps must be taken. Most important is enhancing the feeling of partnership between patient and clinician. In effect, this means establishing a 'therapeutic partnership' between the two as the basis for treatment. To do this it is recommended that methods be employed which engage the patient in the design and implementation of his or her own treatment, and focus on the development of a sense of concordance or agreement, thus enhancing the patient's beliefs about the efficacy and desirability of what is being done. Of course, this entails the clinician spending time listening to the patient and regularly monitoring progress.

As a professionally administered interview, rather than a self-administered questionnaire, the way in which quality of life profiling engages patients in an ongoing therapeutic alliance should be a key benefit to both the service user and the clinician. Patients prefer a full interview and do not object to answering questions (the LQOLP is 100 items and the QLS-100 is the same). The immediate, attractive computerized feedback from analytical support software under development appears to answer successfully some of the objections to quality of life usage cited above.

What is the right length for a quality of life measure?

Various investigators have attempted to identify the appropriate number of individual items for a given domain or total interview. Nagpal and Sell (1985) incorporated Andrews and Withey's findings into their work and concluded similarly that the number of particular concerns or substantive interests exerts a major impact on the coverage of the instrument. The more broad and heterogeneous these interests, the larger the number of items needed in the battery. An equally important consideration is that within an item battery of a given length there is a trade-off between breadth of coverage and accuracy. In designing a measuring instrument, one faces a range of options, from the assessment of many different concerns, with a single item tapping each, to the assessment of a few concerns using many items for each one (Nagpal and Sell, 1985).

The items required in a given scale are governed by a number of factors. Fitzpatrick *et al.* (1992) have identified six specific requirements of quality of life assessments, each of which may determine, in part, the appropriate length of a quality of life measure:

1. Multidimensional construct,
2. Reliability,
3. Validity,
4. Sensitivity to change,
5. Appropriateness to question or use, and
6. Practical utility.

Multidimensional construct

Quality of life is widely regarded as a multidimensional construct (e.g. WHOQOL, 1995). The number of questions required to measure it will vary across domains. In the case of some domains, e.g. religion, there exist a very few questions that explain all of the variance for that single life domain. Religion is predicted by satisfaction with one's particular religion and the frequency with which one is able to practise. This is not true of other areas such as living conditions. No single question appears to exist which will adequately explain satisfaction with living circumstances. Here, underlying opinion appears to be overly diffuse and over determined with several questions being required. Indeed some concepts are really most diffuse. For example, self-concept, mental health, satisfaction with one's living situation, health and social relations are all diffuse concepts with many constituent parts. In respect of multidimensional constructs, the number of questions is greatly determined by statistical necessity. The more questions that are asked, the greater is the probability that one's final rating will approximate the true mean.

Reliability

Reliability refers to errors in measurement and the smaller the degree of error, the more accurate and reliable the measure. A reliable rating scale will be sufficiently robust to remain stable over time. The number of items employed to make a measurement is only one of a number of factors that will influence accuracy. If a rating scale has too few measures of a domain, it may be subject to whim or undue fluctuation, especially in the case of psychiatric patients where one anticipates such fluctuations.

Obviously, within any given research enterprise one must be prepared to acknowledge a conflict of desires. On one hand is the desire to cover a wide range of concerns, in the extreme, perhaps, measuring each with only a single item. In contrast, one may wish to devote many items to covering one area of concern in great detail. Whichever is chosen, each question set will produce a mixture of systematic variance and random variance. What is to be determined, is the essential number of questions which are needed to produce the most accurate set of data.

Validity

Validity can influence the number of questions in several ways. 'The length of the rating scale will be influenced by the similarity of different questions within a domain. Where the questions use words that are really identical in meaning, fewer questions may be necessary to achieve a high degree of reliability or validity. Where the nuance varies considerably between a list of statements, more questions will be necessary due to the variability. However, more "ground will be covered" by the questionnaire' (Research and Education Association, 1981). Different domains are shown to vary widely according to the number of questions required to adequately account for the available systematic variance.

Sensitivity to change or responsiveness

One reason for insensitivity to change is that larger, more generic instruments may include several items not relevant to the particular disease or treatment group. This creates error and masks true change. On the contrary, however, an instrument may equally prove to be insensitive when it is too narrowly drawn, perhaps due to enforced brevity, to tap the 'subtle but important changes in patients' (Fitzpatrick *et al.*, 1992). Equally, too narrowly drawn an instrument, of course, may be reliable but invalid in the sense that it applies to too few cases to be of use. The best guide is probably empirical, i.e. if an instrument tests as having sensitivity, it is not too short.

Appropriateness to question or use

'Form follows function', but is influenced by cultural as well as clinical and organizational context. As this chapter is written, research proceeds into the lives of patients treated under conditions of high security, conducted by the author and his colleagues. Preliminary attempts to revalidate the LQOLP on these patients have met with mixed results. Those patients with severe personality disorders, who have been detained, often because of having committed horrible, callous acts, appear not to respond to these scales as predicted from the results of studies of other patient populations. To measure their quality of life will require a different approach. It may well be that people who do not appear to share the mores of a host culture, who stand outside its values, cannot, nor will not, share their life satisfactions, no matter how sympathetically they are encouraged.

In a different vein, van Nieuwenhuizen (1998) has done extensive research on clinical subjects in the Netherlands. In order to make the LQOLP workable within that context, it was thought necessary to extend it. An extensive user inclusion exercise was carried out employing the concept mapping method. As a result of this research, the Dutch investigators have extended the questionnaire's length to 138 questions, adding a domain on 'life regard' or 'sense of purpose', in order to accommodate their particular cultural and research needs.

At the same time, the LQOLP is also being shortened (Priebe *et al.*, 1999a). A questionnaire (29 items long) has been devised and piloted (which this group are pleased to include in this volume). The Manchester Short Assessment of Quality of Life (MANSA) has been shown to have face, concurrent and construct validity. If properly administered, it can produce information of high quality, quite suitable for inclusion in a minimum data set.

Practical utility

In the realm of practicality, the demands on quality of life scales vary considerably but greater demands are made here than in any other area. Without attempting to exhaust the discussion, the following illustrative points appear to be well supported by reason and experience and will influence the length of a measure.

Clinical factors

Clinical time is expensive. To reduce the amount of time spent on the task of assessment is to increase efficiency. Within UK human service organizations, it seems to be a widely held contention that a long questionnaire must be wasteful of time, even if it is not. Even the amount of time required for scoring a scale must be considered in design. Also, clinical workloads are high. To reduce the amount of time with any one patient allows for better management of a greater caseload.

Patients' conditions must be a concern. Boredom, lack of concentration, and short attention span are three characteristics common to severely mentally ill patients that are exacerbated by long interviews. Fatigue is also an important determinant. For some patients, the length of the interview may be critical. Unlike professionals, they may not be used to sitting and having lengthy conversations. Some patients can become tired and even irritable during a long interview. A questionnaire which contains a greater number of items might be construed as being more intrusive. Coupled with hints of criticism or emotionality, such questioning might contribute to relapse in both schizophrenic and depressive patients. All of these may indicate a briefer interview.

It is important that the question sets are not repetitious. Experience shows that both clinicians and patients are resistant to questionnaires that ask them the same questions repeatedly, or the same questions simply rephrased. Large numbers of inversely worded statements are to be avoided.

The most important determinant from a clinical point of view is that the number of questions does not become a bar to compliance. Having said this, the length of the questionnaire is seldom seen as a bar by the patient (Oliver et al., 1996). Most complaints come from the professionals who administer them. It is reasonable that most patients enjoy talking about their lives to their therapists/key workers. Most importantly, an interview needs to be long enough to allow the patient to feel that his/her concerns are really being taken on board and fully understood.

A quality of life assessment also needs to be an interview. That is to say that it is not simply the most efficient battery of questions. It may need to include questions which are not necessary the scientifically most predictive in order to make the interview comprehensible to the patient. Certain questions must be asked as they are expected and without them one could not ask other questions. 'Do you have friends?' needs to be preceded by 'Are you the sort of person who needs friends?' The two questions may not be of equal weight scientifically, but if both are not asked the patient will only feel compelled to explain. In effect this makes the interview less valid and satisfying.

Data requirements

One parameter that affects instrument design, particularly the length of the instrument, is the method by which data are collected. Andrews and Withey (1976) suggested that face-to-face individual and group interviewing are both appropriate in certain circumstances. Other methods, such as postal questionnaire and telephone interviewing, were markedly less successful and generally not to be recommended. The resources demanded by data collection, processing and analysis are other parameters that must be considered in quality of life instrument design. Service research as an enterprise must be judged alongside competing priorities within health and social care services, like management, education and training and, of course, clinical practice. Underfunded services cannot generally afford very elaborate research and evaluation methodologies. Gathering data and processing it are major sources of costs in evaluation and it is important that methods be efficient, effective and economical. Clear and concise questions, whose answers are easily recorded, coded and entered for analysis are desirable. Especially in the case of mentally disordered patients, questions should not lead to further confusion but should foster clear communications between worker and patient and/or family.

Substantive interests of investigators

The particular interests of the investigator must be a major influence in the design of a questionnaire. Data users with broad interests will require larger batteries of data items. Where a user's interests are more focused data gathering techniques may be applied in a more limited fashion.

In summary, the issues of the appropriate number of questions, in a given life domain or scale will vary according to a number of circumstances. Taking into account the demands of substantive interest, precision and cost, Andrews and Withey conclude that in their own experience using two items to assess feelings about a given concern would be substantially better than just one, three would be somewhat better than two, but rarely would it be worth using more than four items per concern. They recommend that when designing an instrument to assess perceptions of well-being, at least two and possibly three items per concern should be included. Under austerity conditions, just a single item per concern might be used, but, even with substantial resources, rarely would there be a need to use as many as four (Andrews and Withey, 1976).

Also, using concise questions, Andrews and Withey estimated that, among the general population, four or five items can be answered in a minute. From this observation, the size of the battery of questions that can be answered within a given resource can be estimated easily. They made the observation that 'something of potential interest and usefulness can be accomplished in as little as three or four minutes, and by devoting even a modest part (e.g. 10–15 min) of a general purpose survey to assessment of perceived well-being, substantial information can be obtained' (Andrews and Withey, 1976).

This guidance has been followed by several investigators (Nagpal and Sell, 1985; Lehman, 1988; Oliver, 1991a).

Functional approach to quality of life measurement: a brief illustration of instrumentation

In attempting to pull the above discussion together, it is challenging to apply some of the criteria. As an exercise designed to link specific types of

Table 6. Summary: instrument characteristics by function.

Function	Type	Number of domains	Number of items	Completion time
Screening	Interview	1–4	5–20	5–10 min
Surveys	Interview	9–15	65–200+	30–60 min
Audit	Professional rating	1	1–5	1 min
Service outcomes	Interview	9–15	65–200+	30–60 min
Clinical	Interview	9–15	65–200+	30–60 min
Cost analysis	Professional rating	1–4	5–20	5–10 min
Clinical assessment	Interview	9–15	65–200+	30–60 min

scales/measures to specific uses, the following summary table (Table 6) is offered by way of clarification and is intended to act as a focal point for discussion. These should be regarded as suggestions drawn from the literature and experience, and not fully established or empirically derived facts.

Discussion and conclusions

The combination of the number of domains and individual items necessary to capture each is open to debate. To begin with, there is a bewildering variety of instruments, most of which are now being defined as quality of life instruments, largely as they measure some aspect of quality of life or another (i.e. they are domain-specific). Their lengths range from a single question to several hundred with their completion times varying from one minute to a few hours.

Measurements of all lengths and durations can suffer from problems of reliability and validity, and design is frequently a trade-off of one against the other. In the Andrews and Withey research, it was established that 30 or 40 different concerns can each be tapped by several items or as few as six concerns might be tapped by a single question. Andrews and Withey postulated that the number of items required will fall between around 100 and six. The exploration of a variety of valid quality of life interviews which exist seems to support this finding amazingly closely (Lehman, 1996). If each item takes on average 12–15 seconds to complete (Andrews and Withey, 1976), then 100 items will require approximately 20–25 minutes with non-clinical populations and somewhat longer with clinical populations. The five-question scale proposed by Spitzer *et al.* (1981) took on average 1 minute to complete with a clinical population, i.e. 12 seconds per item. Costing and times may be computed accordingly. The number of domains used varies from instruments that are designed to address a single area of concern to those spanning the spectrum of human concerns. Within a truly multidimensional assessment, up to a dozen domains may be covered. Doubtless, there is cultural variability in the content (e.g. Nagpal and Sell (1985) discuss the cultural specificity of a 'transcendence' domain), and domain-specific and health-related quality of life measures are too restricted in their subject matter for many functions.

Accepting these points, the central supposition of this chapter is that provided that it is scientifically sound, one may choose an appropriate quality of life measure according to the function it is to serve. The functions are evolving as human service organizations move to becoming concerned with outcomes and the introduction of scientific measures into the various functions of the organization become more a matter of accepted practice. Certainly, unduly long measures are objected to by clinicians and managers alike but for different reasons. However, the shortest instrument is not always the best, as various authors have concluded. Users are tolerant of lengthy interviews, provided that they do not become bored, etc., or that the interview does not exacerbate their symptoms.

At present, there is too little empirical research on the subject to state precisely which questionnaire is best suited for which purpose, but screening and auditing are two tasks which probably require the briefest measures. On the other hand, population surveys and evaluations of services are more tolerant of lengthy measures especially if they are being administered by paid researchers or the subjects are being paid. It is probably fair comment that a market now exists for quality of life measures and a variety of forms are emerging to define and service those demands. Certainly, more research would be useful to clarify these points.

Whatever choices are made, the clinical state of the patient must be considered in selection. Not only are the patient's symptoms relevant, but so are their interests and aspirations. Determining the scope, scale and facets of a quality of life measure should be guided by the notion of putting the user and his or her predicaments at the centre of consideration. A new technique, 'quality of life profiling' is being developed around the LQOLP, a 35–50 minute interview (100 items). The purpose of this is engagement in clinical practice, and the length and duration of the interview are not generally a barrier to usage for this purpose. A new computerized system to deliver the questionnaire, in either interviewer or self-rated form, provides useful immediate graphic feedback, lack of which is another source of resistance in implementation. This work is still in a developmental stage and use for repeated monitoring and individual programme planning must be approached with some caution until the technique is exposed to more structured study.

4: Discussion

Applying the quality of life construct to clinical practice

FRANK HOLLOWAY

Introduction

This chapter is presented as a response to Joseph Oliver's contribution in this book. It draws on the author's experience as a practising psychiatrist working within a busy British mental health service, an experience that complements that of Oliver, who is a researcher and policy-maker with a social services background (Oliver *et al.*, 1996). The current policy context in Britain is uniquely favourable to the application of structured assessments to clinical practice (Glover, 1995). In response to alarm about the failures of its policy of community care, Government regulation now mandates the regular multi-disciplinary follow-up of all people with a severe mental illness who have been in contact with secondary mental health services (Holloway, 1996a).

Oliver comments on the work of Bowling (1991, 1995). Lehman (1996) has carefully reviewed a wide variety of scales that have been described as measures of quality of life and their possible clinical applicability. Measures are conceptually heterogeneous, assessing 'objective' life conditions (e.g. Malm *et al.*, 1981; Ager, 1990), Health Related Quality of Life (HRQL) (e.g. Heinrichs *et al.*, 1984) and subjective quality of life (Lehman, 1988; Oliver *et al.*, 1996). The ambiguities and complexities of the quality of life concept are apparent in the World Health Organization's definition of (health-related) quality of life. The definition reads 'quality of life is defined as an individual's perception of their position in life in the context of the culture and value systems in which they live and in relation to their goals, expectations, standards and concerns. It is a broad ranging concept affected in a complex way by the person's physical health, psychological state, level of independence, social relationships, and their relationships to salient features of their environment' (WHOQOL Group, 1993). Oliver identifies a persuasive case for one instrument, the Lancashire Quality of Life Profile, as potentially offering a 'clinical tool for the formulation of care plans and a vehicle for engaging severely mentally ill clients in community care'.

Needs assessment: quality of life and care planning

In 1989 the UK Government published a White Paper, *'Caring for People'*, in which it set out proposals for the development of community care services for a range of client groups, including the mentally ill (Secretaries of State, 1989). This included six key objectives for service delivery, one of which was 'to make proper assessment of need and good case management the cornerstone of high quality care. Packages of care should then be designed in line with individual needs and preferences'. The same document introduced the concept of the 'Care Programme Approach'. It was a requirement that from 1991, British Health Authorities had in place 'systematic arrangements for assessing the health care needs of patients who could, potentially, be treated in the community, and for regularly reviewing the health care needs of those being treated in the community' (Department of Health, 1990). In addition, 'arrangements, agreed with appropriate social services authorities, for assessing and regularly reviewing what social care such patients need'. In practice these responsibilities are delegated to the local 'Provider units' (NHS Trusts). The White Paper also makes much of enhancing the quality of life of those in receipt of community care. It catalysed the local development of individual care planning mechanisms for use under the Care Programme Approach (CPA) and the development of needs assessment methodologies (such as the Camberwell Assessment of Need (CAN), Phelan *et al.*, 1995). Subsequently, the UK Department of Health funded the development of the Health of the Nation Outcome Scales (HoNOS, Wing *et al.*, 1996), an abbreviated outcome measure for mental health which it was felt might appropriately be incorporated within the Care Programme Approach assessment and review process.

Despite its importance to policy and practice the concept of need within mental health services is an area of bitter and unresolved ideological dispute (Holloway, 1994; McWalter *et al.*, 1994). Mental health needs assessment methodologies tend to concentrate on clinical problems and needs for care (Brewin, 1992; Marshall *et al.*, 1995a; Phelan *et al.*, 1995) and to rely on the 'expert' views of raters as to the respondent's need status. More 'holistic' approaches have been developed for the needs assessment of people with 'learning difficulties' (Baldwin *et al.*, 1999) and the elderly (McWalter *et al.*, 1994; Barrowclough and Fleming, 1986). These draw on the principles of normalization and attempt to focus on the strengths of service users rather than their deficits.

In a research context, needs assessments could be carried out on a local population of people with mental health problems, identifying deficiencies in the overall service system (see, for example, Holloway, 1991; Murray *et al.*,

1996): the impact of this methodology is, to date, disappointing. There is no evidence that such research has fed back into improvements in the local pattern of care. A needs assessment tool could also form the basis of a care plan (as the clinical version of the CAN is intended to), facilitating the development of a valid list of problems requiring action from caregivers (either informal or professional). It has been argued by Oliver and others (Baldwin, 1986; Holloway, 1994), that subjectively-derived quality of life measures might offer an alternative perspective on care planning which more closely follows the desires and concerns of service users than the narrow 'expert-defined' approach to need inherent in tools such as the CAN.

CAN, LQOL and HoNOS as care planning tools

It is disturbing that in comparison with the literature on quality of life and needs assessment, the scientific literature on care planning is very thin indeed, given that care planning is expected to be the tool through which patients' needs are to be met and their quality of life enhanced. The professional life of many thousands of mental health workers is devoted to, as the current jargon would have it, developing, delivering and monitoring 'packages of care' for people with a severe mental illness, both in hospital (at ward rounds) and in the community (at review meetings). However this activity takes place without the benefit of any significant evidence base, although there is a mass of quasi-theoretical literature surrounding the care planning activities of nurses (Rawlinson and Brown, 1991). It is not even entirely clear that the process of care planning *per se* does any good at all (although evidence of the lack of coherent planning for individuals is apparent in some of the community care tragedies that have occurred in the UK (Petch and Bradley, 1997)). A wide range of *ad hoc* methods of care planning have been developed in the UK to meet the policy demands of the Care Programme Approach (Schneider, J., 1993; McWalter *et al.*, 1994). Official documentation is extremely prescriptive about how the care multidisciplinary plan should be developed and agreed (Department of Health, 1995), but it is silent about what should be included in the care plan, except the mandatory requirement that a full risk assessment (particularly focusing on the risk of harm to others) be carried out (Department of Health, 1994). There is clearly an opportunity for the adoption of structured, validated assessment tools in care planning. The UK Department of Health has funded the development of the CAN and HoNOS. Oliver *et al.* (1996) have reported that the LQOLP has been adopted as 'the first in a library of outcome measures in the Care Programme Approach Support System'.

Table 1 sets out the areas addressed by the CAN (22 domains); the LQOLP (nine domains); HoNOS (12 domains) and The Bethlem and Maudsley NHS

Table 1. Comparison of four care planning instruments.

CAN	LQOL	HoNOS	Local CPA
Day activities	Work and education	Problems with occupation and activities	Day care needs
Education	Leisure and participation		
Benefits	Finances	No	Finances
Accommodation	Living situation	Problems with living conditions	Housing
Intimate relationships	Family relations	Problems with relationships	Family/ relationships
Company	Social relations		
Sexual expression	?	No	No
Physical health	Health	Physical illness	No
Distress	?	Mood disturbance	
Psychotic symptoms	?	Hallucinations and delusions	Mental health
Alcohol	No	Alcohol or drug abuse	
Drugs	No	Cognitive impairment	
Safety to self		Suicidality	
	(Legal and safety)		Risk factors
Safety to others		Aggression	
Home care	No		
Self care	No		
Managing money	No	Problems with	Social
Transport	No	activities of	needs
Telephone	No	daily living	
Child care	No		
Information about illness	No	No	No

CAN, Camberwell Assessment of Need; LQOL, Lancashire Quality of Life Profile; HoNOS, Health of the National Outcome Scale; Local CPA, Bethlem and Maudsley NHS Trust Guidelines for Implementation of the Care Programme Approach.

Trust Care Programme Approach guidelines, which the author was responsible for drafting (seven domains). It can be seen that there is considerable overlap in the areas covered, with the LQOLP particularly strong on areas of social functioning and interpersonal need but either weak or completely failing to address a wide range of 'clinical' needs that are included in the HoNOS and CAN assessments. The CAN is easily the most comprehensive, with items covering the widest range of domains. It does however fail to address potential cognitive difficulties that patients/clients might have. As researchers understand more about the neurocognitive problems associated with psychotic illness, effective treatment planning will have to take this domain into account. HoNOS is reasonably comprehensive, but this comprehensiveness is achieved by conflating quite disparate areas of concern. The

Table 2. Comparison between CAN, LQOL and HoNOS: the nature of the question: items on finances.

CAN ITEM 22
Is the person definitely receiving all the benefits they are entitled to? 0–2 scale (no problem to serious problem)
How much help does the person receive from friends or relatives in obtaining their full benefit entitlement? 0–3 scale (no help to high help)
How much help does the person receive from local services in obtaining their full benefit entitlement? 0–3 scale (no help to high help)
How much help does the person need from local services in obtaining their full benefit entitlement? 0–3 scale (no help to high help)

LQOLP SECTION 6
What is your total weekly income?
What, if any, state benefits do you receive?
About how much more money per week do you need to be able to live as you would wish?
During the past year have you ever lacked the money to enjoy everyday life?
How satisfied are you with how well-off you are financially? 0–7 scale
How satisfied are you with the amount of money you have to spend on enjoyment? 0–7 scale

HoNOS ITEM 10
Rate the overall level of functioning in activities of daily living (ADL) (e.g. problems with basic activities of self-care such as eating, washing, dressing, toilet; also complex skills such as budgeting, organizing where to live, occupation and recreation, mobility and use of transport, shopping, self-development, etc.). Include lack of motivation for using self-help opportunities, since this contributes to a lower overall level of functioning. Do not include lack of opportunities for exercising intact abilities and skills.

0   No problem during period rated: good ability to function in all areas.
1   Minor problems only (e.g. untidy, disorganized).
2   Self-care adequate, but major lack of performance of one or more complex skills (see above).
3   Major problem in one or more areas of self-care (eating, washing, dressing, toilet) as well as major inability to perform several complex skills.
4   Severe disability or incapacity in all or nearly all areas of self-care and complex skills.

CAN, uniquely, identifies the need for information (about the respondent's illness and treatment) as a separate item. Although CAN and HoNOS attempt to address clinical risk (by assessing violence and propensity to self-harm) neither measure appears satisfactory as a risk management tool. The local CPA guidelines are worryingly vague about the areas to be addressed in the care plan.

In addition to the nine life domains assessed within the LQOLP, it includes a measure of general well-being (global subjective quality of life), the Affect Balance Scale (Bradburn, 1969) and Rosenberg's self-esteem scale (1965). The latter two scales might potentially be used as proxy measures, respectively for mood and morale. The issue of morale amongst people with a severe mental illness is both crucial and woefully under-researched, although the impact of severe mental illness on the sense of self has been recognized (Strauss *et al.*, 1989). Despite obtaining data pertinent to these critical issues the LQOLP has however been criticized for neglecting the concerns and values of users by failing directly to address the concepts of empowerment, choice and autonomy that lie at the heart of the current community care ideology (Nocon and Quershi, 1996). The other care planning tools reviewed here provide even less of a perspective on the inner worlds of the service users (although the CAN is able to generate a list of 'needs' solely on the basis of patient/client self-report).

An alternative perspective on these various tools is to look at the nature of the assessments being carried out. The Local CPA guidelines offer no advice on how a particular area in question is to be assessed. It is merely an instruction to consider the area in formulating a care plan. Effective care planning within the Trust is therefore entirely dependent on the success of staff in having identified need in an unstructured way. Table 2 presents items in the CAN, LQOLP and HoNOS relating to the financial situation of the patient/client. The CAN has a separate item about capacity to manage finances, while the HoNOS has a single item covering the whole range of functional abilities ('problems with activities of daily living') which provides no specific information about this particular area of functioning. The LQOLP allows no assessment of functioning in any domain to be made. HoNOS makes no significant attempt to cover the area of financial resources except by implication in ratings of 'problems with living conditions' and 'problems with occupation and activities'. The CAN and the LQOLP contain some attempt to assess the respondent's financial position before going on to address the specific topic of concern for each schedule: the help the patient/client requires to obtain a full benefit entitlement (CAN) and the respondent's satisfaction with their financial situation (LQOLP). An assumption in the CAN is that respondents will be in receipt of welfare benefits. This is accurate for the client group with whom the CAN was developed (people with long-term mental illnesses living in inner city London) but might well not be for other potential client groups of mental health services. However, in common with other needs assessment tools (Holloway, 1994), rating on the CAN triggers specific action (if the respondent is not in receipt of full benefit a need is identified). The LQOLP merely identifies an area of concern for the individual. Both sets of tools operate within strictly defined parameters and it might be argued that in certain crucial ways both miss the point about the experience of suffering from a psychotic illness (Strauss *et al.*, 1989).

HoNOS is designed as an instrument to be readily completed within about 10 minutes by keyworkers (usually nurses or social workers). The CAN can be completed at interview with the client (or, in the research version, with the keyworker) in under 45 minutes as can the LQOLP: an experienced clinician who knows the patient/client well will be able to complete both very much more quickly. One crucial difficulty with HoNOS and CAN is that the quality of the data will vary greatly depending on the knowledge, skills and attitudes of the investigator. As noted above, the judgments demanded in making HoNOS ratings, particularly within 'social' domains, are complex and value-laden. In addition they assume the availability of data to the rater that might be absent (such as their current living conditions). Similar difficulties are apparent in the stem questions in the CAN used to identify 'problems'. Two examples: 'Does the person have any psychotic symptoms, such as delusions, hallucinations, formal thought disorder or passivity?' (item 7: psychotic symptoms); 'Is the person definitely receiving all the benefits that they are entitled to?' (item 22: benefits). The first question requires belief in and an understanding of psychiatric terminology and the availability of an up to date mental state examination. The second requires knowledge of the current benefits system and of the patient/client's current levels of benefit. As mental health services are currently structured, at least in the UK, not all community keyworkers will be competent in the range of need or difficulty encompassed by the measures. One apparent advantage of the LQOLP is that it reflects in a structured way the concerns of the patient/client and thence is less obviously mediated by the viewpoint of the rater. However it has a crucial weakness as a care planning tool: the results of the LQOLP may have little or nothing to do with the stated aims of the care planning process, i.e. meeting the needs of a vulnerable person with a severe mental illness.

The LQOLP and monitoring the outcome of care

Changes at a group level

A key issue for any measure to be used in monitoring the outcome of care is whether it can detect change over time. This author and colleagues have recently carried out a controlled trial of intensive case management against 'standard care' in an inner urban area (Cullen et al., 1997; Holloway and Carson, 1998). 'Standard care' involved treatment by the local service, including community psychiatric nurses with average caseloads of 30, working under the Bethlem and Maudsley Trust's Care Programme Approach policy. The intensive condition consisted of input from a dedicated team with very low caseloads (Waite et al., 1997; Holloway et al., 1996). Outcome was assessed using the LQOLP as well as measures of symptomatology, social performance, social functioning and satisfaction with care. Seventy people with psychotic illnesses identified as 'hard to treat' by local clinicians were included in the study and followed up at 9 and 18 months. Table 3 shows the mean LQOLP scale scores for the population as a whole at entry into the study and at 18 month follow-up. Significant improvements in scores are found for five subscales (work, leisure, finances,

Table 3. LQOLP subscale scores for a sample of severely mentally ill people in a study of community care.

	Baseline	18-month follow-up		Reference mean[a]
Work/education	3.5	4.1	t=2.3 p=0.026 (CI 1.09, 0.07)	4.0
Leisure/recreation	4.6	5.0	t=2.0 p=0.048 (CI 0.85, 0.004)	4.7
Religion	4.8	4.8	t=0.61 p=0.54 (CI −0.20, 0.42)	4.6
Finances	3.4	4.7	t=5.1 p=0.001 (CI 1.75, 0.75)	3.7
Living situation	4.3	4.8	t=2.6 p=0.012 (CI 0.79, 0.10)	4.0
Legal/safety	4.4	4.2	t=0.84 p=0.41 (CI −0.88, 0.36)	4.8
Family relationships	4.6	4.9	t=1.5 p=0.13 (CI −0.12, 0.86)	4.6
Social relationships	4.6	4.6	t=0 p=1.0 (CI −0.42, 0.42)	4.6
Health	4.2	4.7	t=2.9 p=0.006 (CI 0.79, 0.10)	4.4
Mean subscale score	4.2	4.6	t=4.2 p=0.001 (CI 0.79, 0.10)	(4.4)
Global satisfaction	3.8	4.5	t=3.37 p=0.002 (CI 1.17, 0.30)	4.3

[a]Reference mean: quoted in Appendix 2, Oliver et al., 1996.

living situation, and health) with no significant change in four subscales (religion, legal/safety, family relationships, social relationships). Before the study, patients were at or below the published reference mean scores in eight of nine subscales (the exception being religion). At 18-month follow-up mean scores are at or above the reference mean in eight of the scales, the exception being legal/safety, which may plausibly reflect the inner city environment of the study.

Both treatment teams (intensive case management and 'standard care') were attempting to intervene along all LQOLP dimensions except religion and legal/safety (the latter as much an ecological variable as one that can readily be altered). It could therefore be argued that the LQOLP provides data supporting the efforts of the treatment teams (intensive case management and control) in improving the quality of life of their patients/clients, with the exception of the very important 'relationship' dimensions. This failure may reflect lack of activity by care staff in the area: only 1% of case manager time was spent in family interventions and none in activities specifically targeted at enhancing clients' social networks (Waite et al., 1997).

Table 4. Stepwise multiple regression analysis predicting mean LQOLP subscale score.

Independent variable	Multiple R	R^2	F to enter
Beck Depression Inventory $p < 0.0001$	0.53	0.28	20.0
Life Experiences Checklist[a] opportunities subscale $p < 0.0001$	0.70	0.48	23.4

[a]LEC Items: local shops are a short walk away; I travel by car or public transport at least once a week; when I am sick I get to see a doctor easily; I cook meals at least once a week; I can make myself soft drinks or snacks whenever I want to; I do some jobs round the home; I have a pet; I enjoy what I do during the day; what I do during the day is of help or value to others; I am being taught some new skill.

The comparison between the two treatment conditions showed relatively little advantage for the intensive case management team in terms of quality of life (superiority in improving mean total LQOLP subscale scores (all domains summed) at 9 months (ANCOVA $F=5.58$, $p=0.02$) but not at 18 months (ANCOVA $F=1.46$, $p=0.23$)). Other outcome measures showed no difference between treatment conditions, with the exception that the overall satisfaction with care of users of the intensive care services was significantly greater than that of those in the control condition (Cullen *et al.*, 1997). Of direct relevance to the LQOLP outcome results was the finding that case-managed clients were significantly more satisfied with the help they had received for their social problems at 9 but not 18 months. Power calculations indicated that sample sizes of 21 and 44 in each group would be required to detect a difference of one scale point in mean domain-specific perceived quality of life and global subjective quality of life at 95% power. In other words, very large sample sizes are not required in order to detect differences between groups using LQOLP summary measures. These data are broadly supportive of the LQOLP as an outcome measure at a programme level, particularly the use of summary measures (global subjective quality of life and mean domain-specific quality of life).

What do LQOLP scores reflect?

In an attempt to clarify the meaning of the LQOLP scores, a multiple regression analysis was carried out of a range of study measures against the mean subscale score. Having included a wide range of variables, only two contributed to the final regression equation, explaining 48% of the variance in mean LQOLP subscale score: score on the Beck Depression Inventory (Beck *et al.*, 1961) and score on the 'opportunities' subscale of the Life Experiences Checklist (LEC) (Ager, 1990), a normalization-influenced measure of 'objective' quality of life (see Table 4). This analysis suggests that LQOLP data are influenced by both mental state and the respondent's appraisal of aspects of their objective life circumstances. Previous studies have found that ratings of global quality of life within a psychiatrically disordered population are strongly and independently determined by mood (Sullivan et al., 1992; Mechanic et al., 1994; Corrigan and Buican, 1995; Oliver et al., 1995; Holloway, 1996b).

Changes at an individual level

In the case management study understandable changes in life satisfaction within domains frequently occurred. Patient A reported a marked increase in satisfaction about her living situation (from 2.7/7 to 5.2/7) having moved from a hospital setting, which she disliked, to her own flat. Patient B experienced increased satisfaction with his financial state (from 3.7/7 to 6.5/7), having received significant increase in his welfare benefits following engagement with a case management team. However not all responses to the LQOLP are readily understandable. Patient A reported marked satisfaction with her financial state at recruitment to the study (score 6/7), despite being an inpatient and consequently on very restricted benefit. Patient C showed a large shift in satisfaction score for his financial situation during the study (2.5/7 to 5/7) although there was no objective change in his life circumstances over this period. Patient A reported an enormous decrease in satisfaction about legal/safety issues (from 6/7 to 1/7) with no clear-cut explanation (apart from treatment of her paranoid psychosis!). One patient interviewed outside the study, reported complete satisfaction within the religion domain, on the basis of an elaborate psychotic belief system involving Ancient Egypt. This satisfaction was more than balanced by his enormous general dissatisfaction with life based on his belief that his claim to be a British peer was being wrongly dismissed by the Establishment.

Benefits for staff

The views expressed by Oliver in his chapter about the insight that the LQOLP gives to a worker about the concerns and issues faced by the mentally ill can readily be confirmed by interviewing known service users. The bleakness of the lives of people struggling to cope independently with a severe mental illness is quite striking. The LQOLP may provide a powerful training tool to help staff move from a strictly biomedical perspective (although in reality few staff working within community mental health services lack a 'holistic' perspective of their clients' needs). What is less clear is how the individual's dissatisfactions (or even psychotically driven satisfactions) might effectively be addressed without tackling directly the impact of psychosis on morale and cognitive and social functioning. This failure to link the 'health' and 'social' domains of disability reflects the origins of the LQOLP as a care planning tool for mental health social workers (Oliver *et al.*, 1996).

Towards an ideal care planning tool

An effective care planning tool should be based on theoretical understanding of the needs to be addressed within the care plan and evidence of how these needs can most effectively be met. The LQOLP is based on the humanistic principle that everyone shares concerns (as exemplified in the life domains covered). Adopted as a care planning tool it implies that the aim of human services is to maximize the individual service user's life satisfaction within the chosen life domains. It can be argued that this is an inappropriate basis for planning care of individuals with very specific disabilities who, although they share the same aspirations as the general population, have diminished life chances as a result of their disabilities (Holloway, 1994). In addition, psychosis brings with it a different range of life experiences to the general population. These include the pain of psychotic relapse, the loss of hope and self-esteem, the experience of impulsivity and its social consequences, the pervasive nature of the patient role, guilt, the threat to well-being of stressful social situations, social isolation, secondary handicaps of institutionalization and the benefit system and finally the effects of stigma (Strauss *et al.*, 1989).

In contrast to the LQOLP, which derives from a strong theoretical and philosophical tradition within the social sciences, the CAN is based on a rather crude 'shopping list' of potential problems experienced by the mentally ill. Although this reflects consensus amongst 'experts' and service users (Phelan *et al.*, 1995), it has no unifying theoretical basis. A potential basis to underpin psychiatric practice is found in the biopsychosocial model of severe mental illness, which views the 'illness career' of a person with a psychosis as the product of a complex set of interactions between intrinsic vulnerability, psychosocial stressors and toxic environmental factors (such as illicit drugs), pre-existing personal resources and the effects of and individual response to treatment. (See Figure 1 for a simplified and schematic diagram of the biopsychosocial model as applied to psychotic illness.) Within this framework service interventions will aim to maximize the individual's life chances and functioning, leading to the best possible outcome for the individual with the minimum possible reliance on the service system. Care planning will involve assessment of need for interventions that have been shown to improve outcome, with the important proviso that outcome is broadly construed and does not simply represent symptomatology. Such a model would take account of important intervening variables that are often ignored in psychiatric practice, e.g. morale and the effects of stigma. The end result of a care planning tool designed

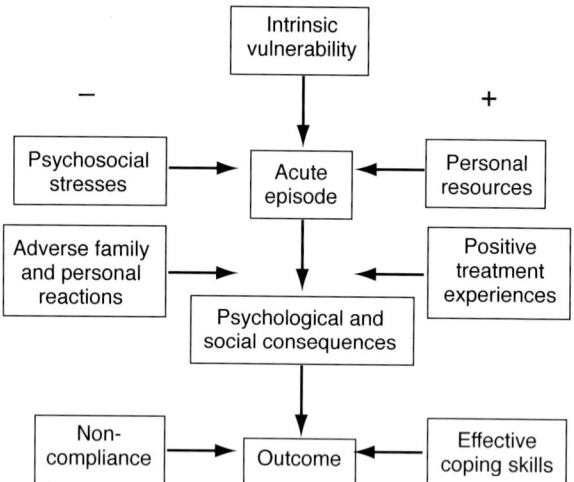

Figure 1. A simplified presentation of the biopsychosocial model of psychosis. Interventions should be targeted at diminishing negative factors and enhancing positive factors acting on the long-term outcome of psychosis.

around this model might well look rather like the CAN, but it would be both more focused towards clinical effectiveness and be, overall, less clinical in tone. It might be linked with treatment protocols and would allow expected outcomes to be generated for each domain of interest. Some issues (for example the effect of stigma) relevant to outcome might best be tackled at a service or even societal level rather than within individual clinical practice. Generally speaking, researchers are a long way from the development of an effective, evidence-based, system of care planning. Perhaps the current debate about the relative merits of tools such as the LQOLP, CAN and HoNOS will prove to have been a modest step on the way towards this goal.

Conclusions

The LQOLP provides an effective tool for measuring the domain-specific and global subjective quality of life of individuals with a severe mental illness. It can be used to monitor the outcome of care for populations in contact with services, and when applied to individual patients, provides a glimpse into their life experiences that is missing in assessments concentrating on mental state. However, the concept of subjective quality of life is too non-specific and limited to be fully acceptable as a basis for care planning. More appropriate would be a tool developed in response to the biopsychosocial model of mental disorder.

5

Neuroleptics and quality of life in schizophrenia

A. GEORGE AWAD and LAKSHMI N.P. VORUGANTI

Introduction

Schizophrenia is a chronic disabling illness, which requires in its management a spectrum of interventions that include psychosocial support, family and individual psychoeducation as well as rehabilitative efforts. However, over the last four decades, the cornerstone of clinical management has been the pharmacological approach. The introduction of the first neuroleptic, chlorpromazine, in the early 1950s and the subsequent development of a long list of neuroleptic medications have profoundly changed the management of schizophrenia and allowed for the shift in management from hospital to community settings. However, the unrivalled role for neuroleptics has been challenged on several accounts, including the increased awareness of the limited usefulness in treating the broader spectrum of psychotic symptoms and the wide range of adverse affects. It is recognized that available neuroleptics can produce a wide range of potentially disabling adverse effects, which can frequently impact negatively on the functional status and quality of life of individuals suffering from schizophrenia (Awad, 1995; Awad et al., 1995a).

The recent interest in quality of life in schizophrenia represents the new image of modern medicine as viewed from a psychosocial perspective. Although interest in quality of life in schizophrenia started in the early 1960s as an extension of the increasing concern about the plight of the chronically mentally ill in the community, following the ill-prepared deinstitutionalization movement, such interests were not sustained for several reasons. Factors that contributed to lack of interest in quality of life studies in schizophrenia have been extensively reviewed elsewhere (Awad et al., 1997c). Such factors included: lack of agreement on a definition of quality of life as well as concerns about the reliability of patients' self-reports, particularly that subjective judgement is a key element of quality of life measurement. As schizophrenic patients frequently experience disturbed thinking and communications, their reports about their inner feelings, values or attitudes toward their medications are often dismissed as unreliable. However, several recent studies, including ours, have repeatedly confirmed the consistency and reliability of patients' self-reports about their satisfaction with medication effects and quality of life (Awad et al., 1995b; Voruganti et al., 1998). Another major factor that contributed to lack of interest in quality of life studies in schizophrenic patients on neuroleptics has been the lack of adequate conceptual models that can allow for the experimental testing of some of the basic aspects of the quality of life concept and its determinants. Fortunately, over the last few years, there has been a serious revival of interest in the concept of quality of life in schizophrenia, particularly related to the introduction of the new generation of neuroleptics. The high acquisition cost of such new neuroleptics compared with the old conventional neuroleptics has brought to the forefront the question of 'value for the money'. Although it is recognized that the component of medications represents a relatively small portion of the total direct cost of management in schizophrenia, yet current financial and budgetary constraints have forced the re-examination of many concepts as cost benefit and cost utility of new versus old neuroleptics. In that context, quality of life in schizophrenia has become an important outcome in clinical trials as well as clinical management. It has also become a tool to compare different neuroleptics, an instrument in decisions about cost and resource allocations as well as an important tool in the marketing of new neuroleptics (Awad et al., 1997a).

The development of an integrative conceptual model for quality of life of schizophrenic patients on neuroleptics

The development of an integrative conceptual model for quality of life of schizophrenic patients on neuroleptics seemed to us an important priority for the understanding of the basic concept, the important factors that contribute to it and, subsequently, to a rational approach towards development of appropriate measures. It is recognized that schizophrenia is a multidimensional disorder that affects multiple areas of functioning such as thinking, affect, cognition and volition. Similarly, its treatment requires multiple approaches including pharmacological interventions, which in turn can produce a wide range of side-effects, some of which can be disabling and impact negatively on quality of life. Our conceptual framework was developed not only to capture the impact of the illness, but also the adverse effects of medication both in manifest presentations such as extrapyramidal symptoms and in subtle forms such as neuroleptic dysphoria and subjective tolerability (Awad 1992, 1995; Awad et al., 1995a, 1997b). According to our model, quality of life is conceptualized as the subject's perception of the outcome of an interaction between three major determinants: psychotic symptoms and their severity, medication side-effects and the level of

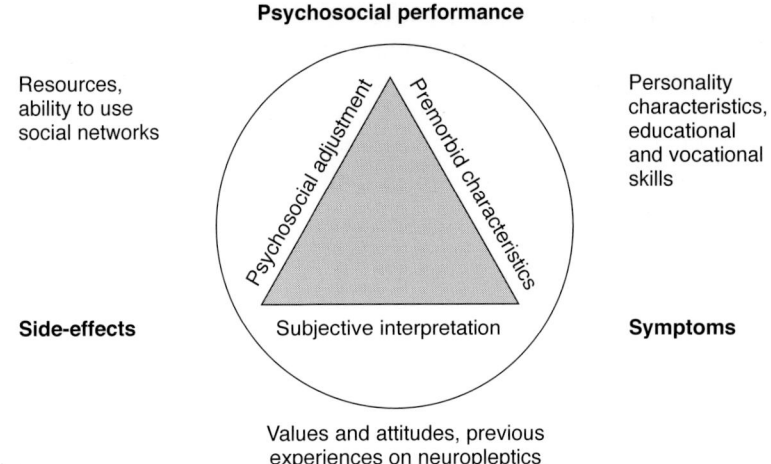

Psychosocial performance

Resources, ability to use social networks

Personality characteristics, educational and vocational skills

Side-effects

Subjective interpretation

Symptoms

Values and attitudes, previous experiences on neuropleptics

Figure 1. Conceptual model for quality of life on neuroleptics (Quality of Life Circle; adapted from Awad, 1992).

psychosocial performance. Other important factors such as personality characteristics, premorbid adjustment, values and attitudes toward health and illness, resources and their availability may modulate such dynamic interaction and impact on outcome. These factors are integrated in a circular model that emphasizes the multidimensional nature of the quality of life concept as well as their interrelatedness (Figure 1).

Details of our conceptual model have been published elsewhere (Awad *et al.*, 1997b). Although our model was initially formulated in the context of providing guidelines for measuring quality of life in clinical trials of new neuroleptics and generally, was clinically intuitive in its development, the value of such models depends on clinical validation and empirical studies. In a series of recent studies, our results broadly endorsed key aspects of the proposed model (Awad *et al.*, 1997b). Multiple regression analysis of the results from a recent study using subjective quality of life as the outcome variable, have indicated that severity of schizophrenia symptoms (partial R^2 = 0.32, $p < 0.0001$) and subjective distress caused by particular side-effects of neuroleptics such as akathisia (partial R^2 = 0.11, $p < 0.01$) and neuroleptic dysphoria (partial R^2 = 0.06, $p < 0.05$), have accounted for nearly half the variance. In another study, although overall a large sample of clinically stable schizophrenic patients displayed a wide range of neurocognitive deficits, their correlation with quality of life was not strong except for a few neurocognitive impairments that had significant correlation (Heslegrave *et al.*,1997b). Reaction time, aspects of the span of apprehension tests as well as iconic memory had significant correlation with subjective quality of life. In all of our studies, this group failed to find any consistent or significant correlation between the dose and the type of conventional first generation neuroleptics and quality of life. On the other hand, significant correlations emerged between several neuroleptic side-effects such as akathisia and neuroleptic dysphoria and subjective quality of life. Obviously, such medication side-effects, although they may relate individually to use of higher medication dosages, can invariably occur unrelated to the dose of medications used.

New neuroleptics and quality of life

Over the recent few years, many new neuroleptics widely described as 'atypical' have been introduced into clinical practice, after a lengthy hiatus, since the introduction of the conventional neuroleptics such as chlorpromazine, haloperidol, etc. The new generation of neuroleptics includes risperidone, olanzapine, and quetiapine and will include others in the near future such as ziprasidone. Clozapine, which is not a new neuroleptic has been reintroduced as an effective pharmacological treatment in situations of treatment refractoriness. Except for clozapine, for which there is good documented evidence for its superiority in treatment resistance, the efficacy of new neuroleptics compared with each other as well as with conventional neuroleptics is generally comparable in spite of some claims that have not yet been adequately and consistently proven. On the other hand, all the new neuroleptics compared with conventional neuroleptics possess a superior side-effect profile and are generally better tolerated by patients. Among the new neuroleptics, as a group, it seems that differences between individual neuroleptics, most likely, lie not in issues related to efficacy, but mostly, to particular side-effects as well as overall subjective tolerability and impact on the functional status and quality of life. So far, only a few studies have systematically compared new neuroleptics with each other as well as with conventional neuroleptics in relation to their impact on quality of life and subjective tolerability (Franz et al., 1997; Meltzer et al., 1990; Revicki et al., 1997; Voruganti et al., 1997). Several studies have already linked subjective tolerability of neuroleptics to compliance, eventual outcome and quality of life (Awad, 1993; Awad et al., 1995b; Browne et al., 1998; Hogan and Awad, 1992; Hogan et al., 1983; Naber et al., 1995; Van Putten and May, 1978; Van Putten et al., 1980).

Preliminary results from one of our recently concluded studies confirm the superiority of risperidone and olanzapine as compared with conventional neuroleptics in terms of side-effect profile, subjective tolerability as well as aspects of quality of life (Voruganti et al., 1997). Using a cross-sectional case-controlled study design for matched groups of schizophrenic patients receiving conventional antipsychotic drugs, risperidone, olanzapine and clozapine, subjective tolerability and quality of life were compared. The subjective tolerability of the drugs was measured with the Drug Attitude Inventory (DAI),

(Hogan and Awad, 1992; Hogan *et al.*, 1983), and Liverpool University neuroleptic side-effects rating scale, (Blyler and Fenton, 1997). Side-effects were quantified by clinicians using Barnes' Akathisia Scale (Barnes, 1989), Abnormal Involuntary Movement Scale (AIMS) (Guy, 1976), and Extra-Pyramidal Symptoms Rating Scale (Chouinard *et al.*, 1980). Global assessment of function was documented for all the patients using the Global Adaptive Functioning Scale (GAF) (Endicott *et al.*, 1976). Quality of life was measured employing the Sickness Impact Profile (Bergner *et al.*, 1981) as modified by Awad (SIP-m) (Awad, 1992, 1995; Awad *et al.*, 1997c) and the Quality of Life Scale (Heinrichs *et al.*, 1984). Patients receiving risperidone and olanzepine scored significantly higher on both subjective measures indicative of positive subjective tolerability. Patients on risperidone, olanzepine and clozapine had better subjective quality of life compared with conventional neuroleptics as measured by SIP-m. However, on the GAF and Quality of Life Scale, improvement in quality of life did not reach statistical significance, which is, most probably, related to possible limitation of both scales in fully capturing the effects of neuroleptics on quality of life in a relatively short-term clinical study.

The choice of a quality of life scale in clinical trials of neuroleptics

In a recent review about measurement of quality of life in schizophrenia (Awad *et al.*, 1997c), our group made the recommendation that any appropriate scale used for measurement for quality of life has to comply with certain requirements:

1. It has to be based on a clear conceptual framework.
2. It has to be specific to the situation and population under study.
3. It has to capture the relevant dimensions of quality of life.
4. The scale has to be psychometrically sound and its psychometrics known.
5. The scale has to include the subjective reports of patients.
6. It has to be 'user-friendly' and not taxing for patients whose functioning has already been compromised by several significant deficits in their mental functioning.

It is our contention that it is preferable to use more than one brief scale to tap different domains of quality of life, rather than loading one scale with a great many items to which most schizophrenic patients will find it difficult to respond. In our studies over the years and particularly with our special focus on the impact of medications on quality of life, our group have employed and contrasted many scales.

It is our experience that a good quality of life scale, appropriate for revealing the impact of neuroleptics on quality of life or for application in clinical trials of new neuroleptics, should be able to capture its pharmacological effects. It should also be sensitive enough to identify minor changes within the relatively short time framework of clinical trials which are usually between 3 and 6 months. The Sickness Impact Profile in the modified short version that this group used in many of its studies, as well as other multicentre studies, has proved to be a suitable scale to capture medication effects on quality of life (Awad *et al.*, 1997b,c). Extensive testing of this shortened modified version has yielded comparable data as reported in the validation of the original scale by Bergner *et al.* (1981). Our data provided evidence for the suitability of the scale for clinical trials of new neuroleptics as well as its sensitivity and reproducibility.

Concluding remarks

Interest in the measurement of quality of life in schizophrenia has been phenomenally increasing over the past few years. However, the wide and increased interest in measurement has not been matched by equal interest in researching several basic issues relevant to the understanding of the concept of quality of life in schizophrenia. The extensive use of neuroleptics in the management of schizophrenia requires a great deal of basic research to reveal the impact of medications, positively or negatively on aspects of quality of life and functional status of the individual. The recent introduction of new neuroleptics coupled with the pressures on the pharmaceutical industry to provide data on quality of life and pharmacoeconomics are creating significant interest in the concept of quality of life on medications and its measurement. The relatively high cost of new neuroleptics has compelled hospitals and drug benefit plans to examine whether such benefits from new neuroleptics can offset the high acquisition costs. Quality of life measurement can be one of those outcomes that reveal differences between neuroleptics and the impact on cost. Quality of life concepts are evolving as a central component in many cost–benefits analyses. On the individual level, improved quality of life of schizophrenic patients can not only reduce their suffering but also return them to a somewhat productive role in life. Clearly, medications alone are not enough to reverse many significant deficits in the schizophrenic illness but the availability of better and more tolerated neuroleptics can contribute to the success of other additional rehabilitative efforts. For the clinicians, the recognition of the various aspects of quality of life of their patients may provide them with opportunities to tailor their management approaches according to the individual's needs. Although symptomatic improvement and control of side-effects seem crucial for successful rehabilitation of schizophrenic patients, for clinicians, shifting their conceptual clinical approach from just symptom improvement to an improved function and quality of life can enhance their ability to help their patients.

5: Discussion

Quality of life assessment: an anthropological perspective

RICHARD WARNER

Introduction

George Awad and Lakshmi Voruganti's chapter on the measurement of quality of life in assessing the impact of different neuroleptic agents highlights an important issue in this research area – the role of subjective and objective measures. Awad and Voruganti take as their starting point the following definition: 'According to our model, quality of life is conceptualized as the subject's perception of the outcome of an interaction between three major determinants: psychotic symptoms and their severity, medication side-effects and the level of psychosocial performance'. Appropriate to that model, they choose as the outcome variable subjective quality of life. Not surprisingly, perhaps, they conclude from their research that a primarily subjective measure, the Sickness Impact Profile, is the most suitable scale in discriminating against the effects of medication. Conversely, they observe that more objective measures, such as the Global Adaptive Functioning Scale and the Quality of Life Scale, failed to reveal significant differences between standard and novel antipsychotic agents.

One needs to examine Awad and Voruganti's starting assumption. One might reasonably suppose that the internal experience of using different antipsychotic medications would be one of the best examples of the value of the subjective reporting of quality of life assessment in medicine. However, let us assume, for the sake of argument, that a novel antipsychotic drug was introduced which produced minimal side-effects but was relatively ineffective in stabilizing the positive symptoms of schizophrenia. In this case, the pharmaceutical company might be pleased with the outcome of a study that emphasizes the subjective experience. However, the user, the family, the community and the psychiatric treatment agency would be ill-served by a study which failed to document objective instability of housing, work and social relations and deficiencies in social functioning and social inclusion.

Can we rely upon the subjective appraisal of such life domains to be accurate?

Subjective and objective data

Researchers studying the quality of life of people with psychiatric disorders often find that patients' subjective satisfaction ratings of different areas of their lives bear little or no relation to their objective life circumstances. For example, the subjective quality of life of patients with schizophrenia in a Swedish study (Skantze et al., 1992) was unrelated to their objective standard of living. Expressed levels of life satisfaction, Barry and Crosby (1996) point out, generally tend to be high regardless of the population surveyed and cannot be used as absolute indicators of life quality. Subjective measures have proven disappointing both in determining differences between subjects in objectively different states and in detecting response to change. Subjective reporting of change is burdened with problems of reliability; the same objective event may result in opposite evaluations from the same person, depending on the person's emotional state at the time of interview (Schwarz et al., 1994). Objective improvements in life circumstances often fail to produce positive changes in subjective satisfaction. In fact, Lehman (1996) reports, interventions that produce objective improvements may lead to a transient *decrease* in life satisfaction as patients become aware of how their lives might be better.

Similarly, objective distinctions in quality of life between samples in different settings or circumstances are often not associated with differences in subjective satisfaction in the same domains of life. Thus, in a comparison of people with schizophrenia in Boulder, Colorado, and Bologna, Italy (Warner et al., 1999), although objective quality of life measures clearly favoured Bologna subjects over Boulder subjects, subjective satisfaction ratings were similar at each site. When a factor analysis was applied to these data, objective quality of life variables sorted separately from subjective satisfaction ratings, suggesting that they measure different underlying constructs.

Psychiatric diagnosis and psychopathology may complicate the picture further. Atkinson and colleagues (1997) observed that subjective quality of life ratings were higher in people with schizophrenia than among those with affective disorder, but that objective measures indicated the reverse – worse quality of life among patients with schizophrenia. These researchers question the value of subjective quality of life measures in people with psychiatric illness since, they conclude, scores may be influenced by affective bias, thought disorder, poor insight and recent life events.

Problems with the lack of correspondence between objective conditions and subjective satisfaction scores are not restricted to people with mental disorder, however; similar conclusions have been drawn from general population studies. Many researchers point out how little demographic variables, such as income, age, gender, marital status, and ethnicity, contribute to subjective well-being in the general population (Diener, 1984). Subjective and objective ratings in the same life domain may be unrelated. Objective ratings of health, for example, show only a weak relationship to overall subjective well-being, although subjective measures of health are strongly associated with well-being (Diener, 1984). Agreement between objective conditions and subjective appraisals declines as the task of appraisal moves from descriptive fact (e.g. frequency of contact with family) to affective evaluation (supportiveness of family members) (Campbell *et al.*, 1976).

The disparity between subjective and objective measures becomes especially problematic when quality of life is used in assessing the effects of treatment. Clinicians and funding agents expect that adequate service provision will lead to improvement in both client circumstances and well-being. However, the two outcomes do not necessarily go hand in hand, and evaluators may be obliged to decide which is more relevant in a given instance; the answer is often not clear-cut. Those who work with the seriously mentally ill recognize that subjective well-being cannot always be the primary goal of treatment, especially in the case of patients in involuntary treatment. On the other hand, agencies operating in the competitive managed-care marketplace, where consumers have considerable power, are likely to give a good deal of weight to subjective satisfaction and well-being measures. As researchers struggle with this issue, dialogue can become difficult. Some researchers are ready to abandon subjective measures (Atkinson *et al.*, 1997) while others, like Awad and Voruganti, hold them to be paramount (Editorial, 1995; Gill and Feinstein, 1994). A conceptual approach known as emics (pronounced as in 'bulimics') and etics (pronounced as in 'aesthetics') from the field of cultural anthropology offers insights which may help restore the dialogue.

Emics and etics

Pike, an anthropological linguist, developed the terms emics and etics, from the linguistic concept of phonemics and phonetics, as a way of discriminating between different types of data which are gathered in the study of cultural phenomena. For Pike, an emic unit of data is something which is regarded by insiders (natives) of a culture as the same entity regardless of etic variation – which an outsider can objectively observe and verify (Pike, 1967, 1990). For example, in the study of language, the unaspirated /p/ sound (as in 'up') and the aspirated /pʰ/ sound (as in 'pull') are identical to speakers of English but not Hindi. The two sounds are phonetically distinct but are phonemically the same in English. Pike extended this concept to non-linguistic cultural events. Thus the Bathonga of Mozambique use the same (emic) kin term for mother and mother's sister although from the biological (etic) point of view these are two distinct relatives. Similarly, a 'hit' in baseball is the same emic phenomenon to fans of the sport, but, to an English tourist, it is etically comprised of a multitude of different types of events.

Harris (1968) modified Pike's emic/etic distinction. In Harris' definition, emic statements refer to logical systems whose discriminations are real and significant to the actors themselves, and etic statements depend on distinctions judged appropriate by scientific observers. Thus far, Harris' definition is similar to Pike's, but the two differ (as shown below) in the way in which they apply emics and etics to the analysis of cultural data. The contribution of the emic/etic distinction to an understanding of the subjective/objective distinction in quality of life research is dealt with in detail elsewhere (Warner, 1999) but the conclusions, drawn from the anthropological research and applied to the quality of life field, may be summarized as follows:

- Subjective appraisals and objective information are different kinds of data. This suggests that composite indices of quality of life using both subjective and objective data are unsound (Muldoon et al., 1998).
- Both types of data are needed. It is important to recognize the independent importance of subjective appraisal of well-being and objective functioning in quality of life assessment (Muldoon et al., 1998).
- Both types of data can be collected from patients. Standard interview schedules and self-report instruments can supply the information.
- It may be necessary to override subjective data to develop a valid predictive model. For example, objective data may reveal changes in patient functioning associated with a switch to a new medication and predict future benefits, while subjective satisfaction ratings show no advantage.
- Objective circumstances should not be expected to predict subjective evaluations of those circumstances or vice versa. Satisfaction measures may decline even when objective circumstances are improving (Lehman, 1996).
- Objective data are particularly important for the prediction of change over time. A psychological adaptation or 'response shift' can occur in chronic illness, as a consequence of which patients' appraisal of their current state shifts; their responses to subjective well-being questions can change substantially, weakening the connection between subjective assessment and objective circumstances (Muldoon et al., 1998). Assessment of the impact of novel treatment methods in chronic disorders, therefore, will require reliance on objective assessments.

Idealism versus materialism

In anthropology, there is controversy, largely between the adherents of Pike and Harris, over the appropriate use of emics and etics. In quality of life research, there is a similar debate over the application of subjective information. In each field, the dispute rests on differing opinions about the basic task of the discipline. For Pike (1967), a cultural idealist, the ultimate locus of reality is within the individual or culture. Therefore, the value of etic data is to provide a starting point for the analysis; the ultimate goal is to replace etic explanation with one that is totally emic. Harris (1979), a cultural materialist, would not deny the emic reality, but, having a pan-cultural view, his goal is the discovery of etic structures which allow one to make general statements about particular cultural events – to describe both emics and etics and, where possible, to explain one in terms of the other.

Similarly, there are quality of life researchers, like Awad and Voruganti, who, in Pike's tradition, consider the individual's perception of his or her circumstances to be the essential reality (Editorial, 1995; Gill and Feinstein, 1994). This approach has the advantage of empowering the consumer by giving him or her a central role in the development of treatment services. Others, like Harris, see the subjective view as an element in building a description of the subject's life and, taking an ecological approach, use the information to establish explanations of quality of life patterns which apply more generally (Muldoon *et al.*, 1998). This approach has the merit of allowing conclusions to be drawn that can benefit a broader constituency. The most practical information for portraying outcomes of mental health services is etic (does the person have accommodation?). However, in order to understand such data and design an intervention to change the outcome, emic information can be very useful (does the person wish to spend his or her income on rent?). For service systems, objective indicators such as adequate accommodation, access to good treatment, and changes in patient functioning may be the most important things to measure. In order to understand why some patients do not accept housing that is offered, do not comply with treatment or choose not to work, subjective measures will be needed. The combination can lead more directly to service improvements that are sensitive to consumers' needs.

Conclusion

It seems important to those providing clinical services and to researchers (like Awad and Voruganti), to ask the customer how one's life satisfaction has been affected by illness and treatment and to place weight on the answers. It also appears that these responses may not necessarily accurately reflect objective circumstances. Conversely, other researchers, frustrated by the lack of correspondence between subjective and objective information, who wish to disregard subjective evaluations should recognize that these data have a place in understanding particular instances, if not in forming predictive models.

Anthropology needs emic data because the discipline 'plays a role as international culture broker' (Lett, 1990). Quality of life researchers need subjective data because their mission includes understanding the inner experience of their subjects. Emic and subjective data are essential to both fields, but it is crucial that both sets of researchers understand how these data may be applied. An appreciation of the distinction between emic and etic data and processes, argues Lett (1990), is essential to all the social sciences.

6

Future research in quality of life in mental health care

ANTHONY F. LEHMAN

Introduction

Research on the quality of life experienced by persons with mental illness is nearing the end of its second decade. The impetus for this research emerged independently at several initial locations, suggesting that it was an idea whose time had come (Lehman, 1996). Once underway, quality of life research on mental health care has spread world-wide. Acknowledging that quality of life research has grown impressively in recent years, it seems timely to take stock of what issues remain and where to go from here.

This chapter raises several methodological and conceptual questions that are pressing with regard to the current state of quality of life assessment and future applications of knowledge about quality of life and mental illnesses. The goal is to present an agenda which ensures that the quality of life research in mental illness does not become a passing fad in the history of understanding and helping persons with mental illnesses.

Should quality of life be a concern of health care systems serving persons with severe and persistent mental illnesses?

In the late 1970s when quality of life was just becoming a research issue in mental health, it was easy to argue that researchers needed to pay more attention to aspects of patients' lives other than symptoms and illness. At that time, there was discomfort with the singular focus on 'clinical' outcomes being the sole measure of effectiveness of health care services. This was not only in mental disorders. Indeed concerns about quality of life were much further along at that point in measuring the outcomes of treatment for other serious medical disorders, especially cancer. It was recognized that parameters such as tumour size and numbers of metastases did not adequately reflect the well-being of the patient. The well-known medical aphorism, 'the operation was a success, but the patient died', was often cited.

The extension of this line of thinking to the care of persons with serious mental illnesses was relatively straightforward. It was becoming clear that symptoms did not bear a direct correspondence to level of functioning, and patients and families often complained that psychiatrists did not listen to their needs and wishes, but rather focused on reduction of symptoms. The rise of quality of life research in mental illnesses actually paralleled the formulation of empirical symptom criteria for various disorders as embodied in the Diagnostic and Statistical Manual of the American Psychiatric Association (American Psychiatric Association, 1980). At the same time, researchers were codifying mental illness in terms of symptoms, thus expanding our concerns beyond symptoms to include quality of life.

Now, nearly 20 years later, most systems of health care face financial crises, and there is tremendous pressure to narrow the mission of health care services. Faced with shrinking resources relative to demand, researchers must again ask whether improvements in quality of life are appropriate goals for health care. It may be philosophically pleasing to speak of quality of life, even good business for competing health care providers to claim they enhance it, but is it reasonable or realistic to focus on quality of life as a health care outcome?

This, of course, is not an empirical question, but one of philosophy and values. There is considerable work currently underway in medical care to develop 'utilities', measures of the relative value placed by persons on various outcomes (Torrance, 1996). For example, one might ask whether it is more important to have treatment that reduces symptoms and the progression of illness at the expense of considerable discomfort, or treatment that ameliorates discomfort but does less to retard disease progression. Such questions are not easy to answer and depend heavily upon the prognosis and the preferences and circumstances of the individual. To the extent that researchers still emphasize individual choice when it comes to health outcomes, it seems that quality of life must remain a major concern of health care. If the point is reached where resources require a more regimented approach to health care outcomes, then the aggregate values of society and the health care industry will take precedence over that of the individual, and quality of life will be less important. Researchers should renew our emphasis on individual choice with regard to health outcomes and hence of quality of life as an important outcome in health care (Lehman, 1995a). Having asserted this, on the empirical side, research into utilities and preferences for alternative outcomes should proceed to help us better understand what people want.

What aspects of quality of life should be of concern in mental health care and research?

Having staked out a renewed philosophical position in favour of quality of life as an important mental health care outcome, there remains the practical issue of what aspects of quality of life are relevant to mental health care research. It is evident that quality of life encompasses a broad range of issues, and it can be fairly argued that health care cannot possibly affect all of these aspects. Indeed, it is grandiose to think so. There is however a realistic tension between those who would argue that quality of life outcomes ought to be narrowly defined in health care and those who argue for a broader view.

The heart of this debate relates to the differences between acute, time-limited health conditions and chronically disabling ones. For the former it seems appropriate to hold health care accountable for those aspects of quality of life that are immediately affected by illness and treatment. For example, in considering the treatment of an acute episode of major depression, it is reasonable to expect the care plan to consider, in addition to depression symptoms, such quality of life issues as short-term impacts on employment and family income and medication side-effects. One would expect the treatment plan to consider how to help the patient return to work as quickly as possible and perhaps how to help the patient and family access short-term disability income payments to cover family expenses during the episode. The treatment plan would also be expected to adjust medications to deal with such side-effects as constipation and impotence. Attention to these kinds of health-related quality of life problems makes the treatment far more relevant to the individual than a treatment plan that measures success by reduction in depression symptoms only. Researchers would not expect the treatment plan to help the patient find a better job or the family a bigger house nor would they expect the plan to help the patient find a spouse. Such long-term quality of life concerns are not in the purview of treatment for an acute episode of illness.

The issues for chronically disabling conditions are very different. Persons disabled by such conditions as schizophrenia, who are unemployed, socially isolated, and have difficulty getting along in society pose a special challenge for society and for health care. Society typically has looked to the mental health care and social welfare systems to provide for the basic needs of the disabled. There is an inevitable blurring of health and social needs. Historically, mental health care systems have provided not only psychiatric and medical care to such persons, but have provided housing, social supports, financial supports, and so on.

Converging on this tradition are two forces that require a careful reappraisal of this situation. First, pressures to reduce health care costs are encouraging health care providers to shift the costs of providing for the social needs of the mentally disabled to other agencies, typically social welfare and criminal justice agencies. There may be little incentive to promote continuity of care across these institutional boundaries. Indeed it may be in the financial interest of the health care provider to do just the opposite. These incentives are certainly true for the competitive managed care organizations in the United States, but may hold equally well for purchasers under single payer systems in other countries.

A second force testing the appropriateness of broad quality of life perspectives on the mentally disabled is the self-help or empowerment movement among mental health care users. Expecting the mental health care system to take responsibility from broad aspects of the patient's quality of life may be reviewed as paternalistic or authoritarian. What business is it of the health care provider how the patient chooses to live?

These points lead to a series of recommendations about future quality of life research strategies and directions. First, as the economic crises in health care seem to overshadow most other issues, it is vitally important for research to evaluate the impacts of the rapidly changing economics and structure of health care systems on patient quality of life. Secondly, it is essential that quality of life research methods retain as their core the patients' concerns. To accomplish this patients must be involved in a variety of ways. At the very least they must be the primary respondents for quality of life assessments. In addition, focus groups can be used to review existing quality of life measures with patients/users to determine if their content and form reflect users' quality of life issues. Finally, patients may directly collaborate in the design and implementation of quality of life research studies.

Subjective versus objective quality of life

What weight should be applied to these? It is quite well known and has been repeatedly demonstrated that the so-called objective and subjective aspects of quality of life are not highly correlated. For example, income typically does not predict life satisfaction (Andrews and Withey, 1976). The maxim, 'you can't buy happiness' seems to hold. Most researchers also seem to view the subjective aspects of quality of life as central to the concept (Spilker, 1990). Otherwise one is left with measures of functional status and standard of living. There is little problem with this bipartite notion of quality of life when objective and subjective quality of life more or less correspond. For example, studies showing patients reporting greater life satisfaction when out of the hospital than when in it provide a consistent picture and little conceptual dissonance. The picture, however, is more confusing when objective quality of life conditions and life satisfaction do not point in the same direction. There are numerous examples of this. This author's research has found that schizophrenic patients, though functionally more impaired, express somewhat greater life satisfaction than do depressed patients (Lehman, 1983a). Other authors have found the same thing (Atkinson et al., 1997; Oliver et al., 1996). Similarly, this group has found that African–American patients report lower incomes and rates of employment, but somewhat greater life satisfaction that do Caucasian patients (Lehman et al., 1995a). What can be drawn from these findings?

They raise two issues. The first, dealt with later, is to question the validity of life satisfaction as a useful outcome as well as the methods used to measure it. The second is how to weigh these two types of quality of life measures in determining the value and effectiveness of interventions. Is it better to have a treatment that makes a person feel better, but does not change how they function or one that makes them feel worse, but improves their functioning and status? This brings us back to the earlier issue of utilities and preferences. If researchers are to adhere to the philosophy underlying quality of life research that the goal is to address the patient's well-being as judged by the patient, then studies should be conducted that examine the trade-offs patients would make on the objective and subjective aspects of quality of life. Similar studies are needed on healthy samples.

Can persons with mental illness provide reliable and valid assessments of their quality of life?

A gnawing issue in the assessment of quality of life for persons with mental disorders is whether persons with mental illness can provide truly valid assessments of their quality of life. On a general level it can be argued that psychometric studies of the validity of quality of life measures for persons with mental illness have produced positive results (Lehman, 1996). That is, these have tended to support the construct, predictive, and criterion validity of quality of life measures. On a philosophical level, it may be argued that to consider quality of life self-assessments of persons with mental illness as suspect or invalid is to invalidate them as people; 'they don't know any better'.

Still, these issues frequently arise when quality of life findings do not coincide with investigator or societal expectations or logic. Researchers must assume that there is something to this concern. As mentioned earlier, it is not known whether disorders of mood substantially affect the level of life satisfaction. Mood may also affect self-assessments of functional status. For example, a depressed patient may report low life satisfaction and cognitively distort and underestimate prior work achievements. Conversely psychosis on average is only modestly related to level of life satisfaction (Atkinson et al., 1997; Lehman, 1983b; Oliver et al., 1996), probably because the effects of psychosis on life satisfaction depend upon the nature of the psychosis. By definition, psychotic persons may distort the reality of their level of functioning. How can this problem be dealt with? Studies are needed to examine in more detail the relationship between quality of life judgements and psychopathology. A variety of research questions can be raised. How does a person's rating of their quality of life vary when they are and are not experiencing major symptoms? That is, holding objective life circumstances constant, how does life satisfaction vary with symptoms? If it does vary, how should this affect the timing of collection of life satisfaction assessments? Holding symptoms constant how does life satisfaction vary across time as changes occur in objective life circumstances? Does psychopathology override the impacts of actual life circumstance changes on life satisfaction? Does depression dampen the effects of improvements in objective life circumstances? Does psychosis distort changes in life satisfaction related to changes in life circumstances? For example, is it necessary to see expected changes in housing satisfaction among the homeless who are psychotic when they achieve decent housing? Many of these questions could be answered from reanalysis of existing data sets or from longitudinal studies that concurrently assess psychopathology, life satisfaction, and objective life changes.

Is quality of life a state or a trait?

A recent study suggests that there may a strong hereditary component to 'happiness'. These investigators found intraclass correlations on a measure of subjective well-being in the range of 0.44–0.52 among monozygotic twins, whether reared together or apart, contrasting with correlations of –0.02— 0.08 among dizygotic twins. Hence it must be asked, 'Is quality of life a state or a trait?'. In contrast to the prior questions about the impacts of current mental status (a state) on subjective well-being, this question asks whether life satisfaction is primarily a function of enduring personality characteristics. In essence, are people inherently optimistic or pessimistic and is this the main determinant of life satisfaction? Again, this question should be examined through longitudinal studies to determine whether and how life satisfaction changes as circumstances change. Do people have an internal set point for life satisfaction to which they tend to return despite changes in life circumstances? How should this be incorporated into ongoing quality of life research? Some data suggest that such enduring temperament characteristics may affect measures of general life satisfaction more than measures of domain-specific life satisfaction, such as housing or job satisfaction (Drake et al., 1996; Lehman et al., 1986, 1991).

How can quality of life be measured in a culturally sensitive manner?

All would agree that quality of life judgements are personal and individualistic. It seems clear that quality of life judgements will be affected by culture and the prevailing ambience within which one lives. This is most evident when trying to translate a quality of life measure from one language to another. The words to describe feelings of life satisfaction may carry substantially different connotations in different languages and direct translations may substantially alter their meaning. Even within the same language, cross-cultural translations may be necessary. An excellent example has been the adaptation of the Lehman Quality of Life Interview into the Lancashire Quality of Life Profile (Oliver *et al.*, 1996). What worked in the United States did not apply as well to the United Kingdom. Cross-cultural problems in applying quality of life assessments can occur between subcultures in the same country. For example, the question, 'How often to you engage in a hobby?' is readily understandable by middle class respondents, but may not be relevant or understandable to impoverished persons. Similarly, questions about leisure activities are quite important to the working middle class, but irrelevant to many homeless persons. If researchers are to use the same quality of life measures cross-culturally, it is essential to conduct careful literal and contextual translations.

How useful are quality of life assessments?

Evaluating intervention outcomes

The major hope in the development of quality of life measures for persons with mental illness has been that these measures will elucidate the impacts of alternative interventions on quality of life. It is fair to say that, at this point in time, quality of life is largely viewed as a secondary outcome, usually after clinical status measures and other more 'objective' measures. I would cast this in a somewhat different vein. It is useful to think of models of outcomes that identify 'proximal' and 'distal' outcomes. (Lehman, 1996). Proximal outcomes are those that most directly relate to the mechanism of action of the intervention and that occur most close temporally to the intervention. Distal outcomes are those 'downstream' from the intervention both in terms of casual mechanisms and time. Hence a new antipsychotic agent may proximally reduce symptoms and cause certain side-effects. The distal impacts on quality of life will be a function of both of these proximal effects. Many similar examples can be presented.

Comparing groups

Some of the earliest studies of quality of life among the mentally ill compared different groups cross-sectionally (Lehman, 1996). These studies found differences between patients in and out of the hospital, depressed and non-depressed, and so on. Such comparisons are useful and it does appear that quality of life measures discriminate between groups quite well. A remaining issue is whether these cross-sectional comparisons inform us about how quality of life may change over time within groups, for example as patients move from the hospital to the community.

Assessing patient needs

One of the more promising applications of quality of life assessments is their utility for assessing patient needs. It is important to know how patients feel about various aspects of their lives in order to identify those areas that cause them the most concern. A major contribution of quality of life assessments to the quality of care may be in structuring a careful inventory of multiple aspects of patients' lives in order to prioritize interventions. Excellent examples of this application from Oliver and colleagues have been quoted earlier in this volume.

Measuring change

Concern remains that quality of life measures are not sensitive to change. This concern is raised when investigators fail to find predicted changes in quality of life. This concern is in part related to some issues already discussed about whether quality of life assessments are overly influenced by psychopathology and whether they are more trait than state. Quality of life measures are more vulnerable to this criticism because they are less understood than certain other outcome measures, e.g. symptoms or work status, and because they are more suspect for all of the reasons previously mentioned. Researchers need more work on understanding how quality of life assessments change in order to decide if they are appropriate change measures in different circumstances.

Planning services

An extension of the application of needs assessment of the individual patient level is the use of aggregated quality of life data to plan the service priorities for a service system. The chapters by Oliver and Warner and colleagues in this volume provide excellent illustrations of work in this area.

Conclusions

Over the past two decades, research on the quality of life of persons with mental illness has blossomed. With this success, the field now faces a series of important questions about the methods that have developed to date, the interpretation and validity of quality of life information, and its utility research and service delivery applications. This stage of thoughtful criticism should be met with interest and enthusiasm. It is vital that critical questions be addressed forthrightly in order to ensure the ongoing vitality of this area of inquiry and its continued development.

6: Discussion

Research in quality of life in mental health care: aims and strategies

STEFAN PRIEBE

Introduction

Research papers frequently conclude with a remark that further investigation into the subject in question is needed. Regarding quality of life in mental health care, one could probably draw up an endless list of questions which might be worth addressing in further research and of methods that may be applied and might yield interesting findings. Such a list, however, would not be too helpful and priorities have to be set, because resources are limited and because research in this area should focus on issues that are most relevant for improving mental health care.

Lehman in the preceding chapter identifies such priorities and outlines areas of special practical and research interest. What follows in this chapter is a string of other ideas, which are not necessarily related. They will address conceptual and methodological issues, experimental research and the relevance of quality of life measures for the therapeutic process.

The function of the construct

This book begins with a chapter on the concept of quality of life. What constitutes quality of life in people with mental illness, remains a central question to many researchers and practitioners. According to constructivism, quality of life may be regarded as a construct, which is intended to enable mental health care to define and fulfil its role in society. In constructivism it does not matter whether a construct is right or wrong, and the relevant question is not whether a given concept of quality of life is correct and reflects 'true' reality. What matters is whether the construct is useful to clinicians, researchers and other people involved in mental health care, and whether it fulfils its purpose. Lehman points out that the reason for introducing the quality of life construct in mental health care was to define aims, and subsequently to assess outcomes. Why is improving patients' quality of life or maintaining it on as high a level as possible a central aim in mental health care?

Aims are based primarily on values rather than arguments or rationales. As has been pointed out in previous chapters, dissatisfaction with more confined conventional aims, such as reduction of symptoms or prevention of relapses, was one of the reasons to go for a more global concept like quality of life. The underlying value is embedded in a certain ideology and Weltanschauung which may be challenged. For instance, several religions, including those of some Christian churches, might argue that a person's quality of life after death is far more important than the quality of life before death, and that the latter is, therefore, the wrong target for concerted efforts and actions in society. In ancient Sparta, the quality of life of the whole community was of a greater value than that of an individual. Thus, defining an individual's quality of life as an aim for health and social services, has cultural, social, political and religious roots, and may be subject to trans-cultural differences and to change over time. The current prevailing concept of quality of life seems to fit well with enlightenment, post-modernism and capitalistic ideology. It goes without a metaphysical dimension; it looks directly and exclusively at individuals and not at communities; it widely neglects the past and the future, focusing on the here and now; it follows individual preferences and tends to avoid the positive definition of other ideologically-based and socially accepted values.

Interdisciplinary research by psychiatrists, historians, sociologists, and philosophers may lead to a better understanding of the various factors determining and influencing the function of the construct of quality of life. Mental health professionals involved in this research would have to look at mental health care from a bird's eye view: their professional behaviour and attitudes would be the subject of their own research. Despite that overlap of the roles of researcher and researched subject, such research might help to clarify the exact task of mental health care in our societies at the current time. Furthermore, one might be able to extrapolate the findings to the future and have some vague notion of which changes are to be expected under which political, economic and social developments. For example, will decreasing financial resources for mental health care undermine the popularity of the quality of life concept, because an improvement in quality of life is unlikely to be achieved for most patients by poorly staffed and poorly resourced services? Or will, on the other hand, less money for mental health care increase the popularity of the quality of life concept, because it gives a relativistic perspective and removes values that are set by politicians and clinicians? Values and aims in mental health care have changed substantially within the last two centuries, and they are most likely to keep changing in the future. Researchers may be experiencing significant changes at the moment, possibly due to diminishing economic resources, different prevailing political ideologies, or just the zeitgeist. The suggested research would have to investigate variations over time and across nations. Does mental health care pursue the same goals in different countries? It seems obvious that there are major differences, which may affect the priority that is given to quality of life as an aim and to the understanding of the concept. An analysis of those differences seems important in order to avoid inappropriate generalization of results from one country to another, e.g. from developed countries to developing countries.

Specificity of the construct

A construct can only be useful if it presents a meaning that is clear and distinct from that of other constructs. Lehman mentions the tension between those who argue that quality of life ought to be narrowly defined in health care and those who argue for a broader view. There are obvious dangers in defining quality of life too narrowly, but there also is a risk of diluting it. If quality of life is to represent the overall aim for mental health care and, subsequently, the ultimate criterion for evaluation, and if it is to include all aspects that might theoretically be associated with good or poor life, it may lose its usefulness. If the criterion of usefulness is not considered, it would be easy to argue that the quality of life concept should incorporate aspects such as meaning of life, personal growth, happiness and fulfilment of life goals. Furthermore, that it should be equally applicable to different individuals, e.g. to a miner, a professional football player or a monk, and to different cultures, and that it assesses disadvantages across different physical and mental illnesses. If, however, the usefulness of the concept is taken into account, some of those demands look less relevant. The professional background of the authors of this book is in mental health care in western industrialized countries. Their main interest may be to define the aims of mental health care and to improve the situation of people with mental illnesses in these countries. In order to achieve these goals, it seems less relevant that the same concept is appropriate for assessing the quality of life in people with somatic illnesses living in very different cultures and social circumstances. Thus, the quality of life concept may be specific, and finding concepts that are useful for a given purpose may be more important than looking for an overall, ultimate, and eternal concept of quality of life.

To be useful in mental health care, the quality of life concept must have an identifiable meaning that is clearly distinct from the meaning of other concepts. There are other concepts than subjective quality of life that are used as subjective evaluation criteria in mental health care, i.e. criteria that are based on subjective statements made by the patients, and that are frequently used for evaluation. These are self-rated psychopathology, self-rated needs, and patients' satisfaction with or assessment of treatment. In a cross-sectional study, all four criteria were assessed in different samples of patients with schizophrenia and with alcoholism using identical instruments (Priebe et al., 1998a). The four criteria showed substantial intercorrelations except for assessment of treatment in acute treatment groups. One general factor explained around 50% of the variance for all criteria in each group, and each of the four criteria contributed to the variance of that factor. It may be concluded that the four criteria overlap in different patient groups and that similar constructs may be assessed under different labels, i.e. that self-rated needs, subjective quality of life, etc., to some extent reflect the same dimension of subjective appraisal. Results of longitudinal studies have so far been less conclusive. Thus, it remains to be seen in which way the different subjective evaluation criteria co-vary over time and in which way they differ in their sensitivity to change. Regardless of longitudinal associations, there is substantial overlap, and a better theoretical framework is required to explain the relationships of and differences between subjective evaluation criteria. Developing that framework, however, requires a wider basis of sound empirical results than is currently available. Further studies might benefit from combining quantitative and qualitative methods for generating and testing hypotheses about the specificity, usefulness and relationship of different constructs.

Another conceptual issue is mentioned by Lehman, i.e. the important association between satisfaction ratings and psychopathology. The literature suggests that depressive symptoms are particularly influential, not only in depressive samples, but also in schizophrenia patients. Dissatisfaction and depressive symptoms have been found to be associated in cross-sectional studies, and to co-vary over time in longitudinal studies (Priebe et al., 1999a). This resembles findings in the general population in which depressive mood also demonstrates a correlation with satisfaction ratings. What remains to be studied, is, first, whether this is due to a one-dimensional correlation and, secondly, whether depressive symptoms influencing ratings are the same in different groups or whether one deals with qualitatively distinct phenomena of depressivity/depression in different samples. Which depressive cognitions are most closely associated with a higher degree of dissatisfaction, and how can those cognitions be specifically assessed? Is there a certain degree or quality of depression influencing satisfaction ratings so much that the latter cannot be usefully interpreted anymore? Existing data suggest that depression is associated with less satisfaction, but that depressive patients still distinguish between different life domains and that they are not equally dissatisfied across all life domains. Moreover, the shared variance between psychopathology scores – including mood assessments – and subjective quality of life is rarely greater than 30% (Kaiser *et al.*, 1997). Thus, although satisfaction ratings are associated with depression, they are a parameter on their own and are not predominantly explained by psychopathology. The construct of depressive cognitions, including negative views of one's self and of the world, needs to be separated from that of subjective quality of life, although the two may be correlated or overlap.

In reformulating the theoretical foundation, it may be necessary to define quality of life much more narrowly than thus far in order to make it clearly distinguishable from other constructs such as needs or happiness. If such a distinction cannot be achieved, the construct of quality of life might have to be given up or merged with other constructs, possibly leading to the development of a new and more global concept of subjective appraisal. The analysis and comparison of several constructs may also assist in avoiding the risk that shortcomings of the quality of life concept might lead researchers to opt for another concept prematurely, e.g. needs, the theoretical foundation of which is even less clear (Heinze and Priebe, 1995; Hoffmann and Priebe, 1996).

Different perspectives

There is a distinction between objective and subjective indicators of quality of life. This terminology refers to the way data are assessed: some data are – at least in theory – objectively assessable and are therefore called objective. Frequently, all observer ratings are termed objective although they involve the subjectivity of the observer. Information, such as the patient's income or his/her place of birth, is regarded as objective because the assessment should be objective and independent of anyone's personal influence. In other words, there is one and only one correct response, which could be checked. So-called subjective data are statements reflecting patients' feelings and judgements and include all self-ratings. This distinction is conventional although, in practical terms, assessment of so-called objective data is also based on patients' statements, and, for example, interviewers rarely check with the tax office whether patients' reports of income are correct or not.

In addition, there is a distinction between assessment of data and interpretation of those data. There may be various perspectives as to which data constitute an index of quality of life, and each perspective is subjective by nature. Whether level of income, depression scores or satisfaction ratings – to name just a few options — are regarded as measures of quality of life is a matter of interpretation. Patients, clinicians, carers, or politicians may have very different views on what they take as quality of life indicators, and nobody can claim the copyright for the one and only definition of quality of life.

The two levels – that of assessment and that of interpretation – are often confused. For example, many scales assessing potential indicators of quality of life are called 'quality of life scales' or something similar, with the term quality of life in the title. Hence, the scale names suggest that the data obtained do reflect quality of life independent of the interpretation. Readers who are not familiar with the scales themselves and with the enormous differences between them may be startled by contradictory results and find it hard to distinguish between issues of measurement and issues of interpretation. An alternative might be to restrict the term quality of life to the level of interpretation. Subjective quality of life as assessed in the Quality of Life Interview, the Lancashire Quality of Life Profile or the Manchester Short Assessment of Quality of Life may be termed satisfaction ratings – a term that is clear, understandable and rarely disputed. Whether those satisfaction ratings, or other data, are regarded as quality of life indicators in the given circumstances, would be a matter of interpretation by whoever uses the measures. The issue of whether a given scale 'really' assesses quality of life would be replaced by whether the scale is a useful indicator for quality of life for the given purpose.

Regardless of whether the terminology will be changed or not, a distinction between these two levels, i.e. assessment and interpretation of data, seems essential for further research. Specific studies may investigate what patients, relatives, professional carers, health services managers, commissioners, health politicians, the general population, etc., deem useful indicators of quality of life, no matter how those indicators are obtained and whether they reflect objective or subjective data. Views as to what constitutes quality of life may change over time depending on the purpose and circumstances of the judgement. A focus on different perspectives of quality of life may replace a desire to yield scores intended to have a similar meaning across all perspectives. Moreover, it would individualize the quality of life concept in two ways: first, the concept applies to an individual life, i.e. that of a person with a mental illness and, secondly, it reflects an individual person's definition and construct of quality of life, i.e. patient, carer, politician, and so on.

New methods for assessing quality of life indicators may have to reflect specific perspectives. As far as patients' own subjective perspective is concerned, there is a demand that scores should be valid, i.e. reflect patients' 'true' satisfaction with life. Since there is no external criterion for validity of satisfaction, the validity of such satisfaction ratings is difficult to assess. The terms objectivity, reliability, and validity of measures stem from psychological test theory. They apply when a test assesses a construct which is clearly defined and for which there is an external criterion for validity. In subjective quality of life, psychological test theory hardly applies at the present since the construct remains unclear. To overcome this problem, it has been suggested that patients' satisfaction ratings should be regarded simply as statements and as verbal or rating behaviours that are valid in themselves as long as they are correctly documented (Priebe *et al.*, 1995). Patients' statements would be analogous to a vote in an election which as such is important and not questioned for its validity, no matter whether it reflects the voter's 'true' political interest. It has not been suggested that this is the only or best way to look at subjective quality of life scores, rather that it is one way of overcoming current conceptual shortcomings.

Analysing and reporting quality of life data

Subjective quality of life ratings may yield simple scores. It has been argued that such scores are inadequate and do not reflect the complex processes leading to a higher or lower degree of satisfaction in the patients. That may be correct. Yet, concept and scores must be useful in mental health care. An analogy to physics might illustrate this: a thermometer is not able to reflect the complex processes and factors determining the climate and influencing variations of the temperature. Thermometers do, however, show one simple score that is highly relevant for action, e.g. how to dress or how to adjust the heating. In mental health care, psychopathology scores are often used similarly. The total scores of the Hamilton Rating Scale for Depression or of the Brief Psychiatric Rating Scale do not reflect the social and intrapsychic processes leading to improvement or deterioration of symptoms. Nevertheless, they can tell the clinician and the researcher very useful information. Thus, the complexity of the construct of quality of life does not necessarily mean that complicated methods for assessment have to be applied or that simple scores have to be avoided.

For reporting data, further simplification might be useful. In many currently used quality of life scales, satisfaction is rated on seven point scales with 1 as the negative and 7 as the positive extreme. Results are usually reported in means (or medians). However, what do such scores tell the clinician or commissioner of mental health services? For example, when a mean score in a patient sample changes from 4.4 to 4.7, does that impress the non-researcher, even if the difference is statistically significant? If the information was condensed and scores dichotomized, one may get percentages of only two groups: patients who are satisfied in the given life domain and patients who are not. Reporting data in such a way may be more clinically appealing. In the following example, both ways of reporting are compared: 408 schizophrenia patients in three groups, 90 first-admitted patients (Priebe *et al.*, 1999a), 175 long-term hospitalized patients Hoffmann *et al.*, 1997; Priebe *et al.*, 1996), and 143 outpatients in community mental health services were assessed using the Berliner Lebensqualitätsprofil (Priebe *et al.*, 1995),

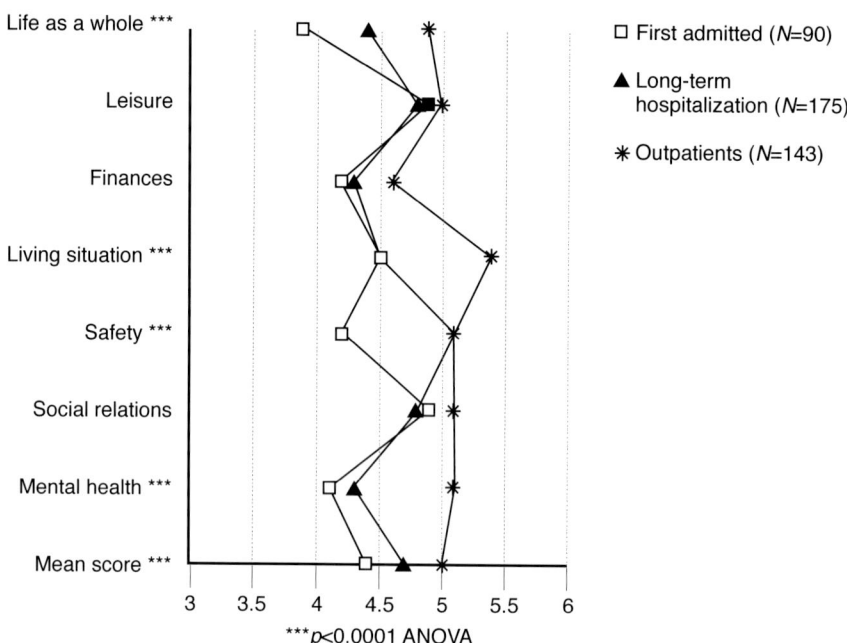

Figure 1. Mean satisfaction scores of three samples of patients with schizophrenia.

the German version of the Lancashire Quality of Life Profile (Oliver *et al.*, 1996). Figure 1 shows the subjective quality of life ratings in the usual way, reflecting means. Differences between the groups in satisfaction with life as a whole, with living situation, safety and mental health as well as in the mean satisfaction score were statistically highly significant (ANOVA, each $p < 0.001$). Figure 2 shows, based on the same ratings, the percentage of not satisfied patients in each group. Statistical tests demonstrate significant differences in the same ratings (χ^2-tests, $p < 0.01$ for safety, $p < 0.001$ for other domains) as the analysis of variance does. Additionally, there is a significant difference in satisfaction with finances ($p < 0.05$) which, however, disappears after Bonferroni adjustment. Changing the cut-off point on the satisfaction ratings for defining the two groups did not produce very different results. Thus, despite the simplified way of reporting the findings, for most of the comparisons the same significant results are revealed.

Yet, only the analysis of variance, which uses means and standard deviations, provides a simple procedure to control for the influence of other factors. In the aforementioned study, when age and the degree of psychopathology, as assessed on the Brief Psychiatric Rating Scale (Overall and Gorham, 1962), are used as covariates in the analysis of variance, the

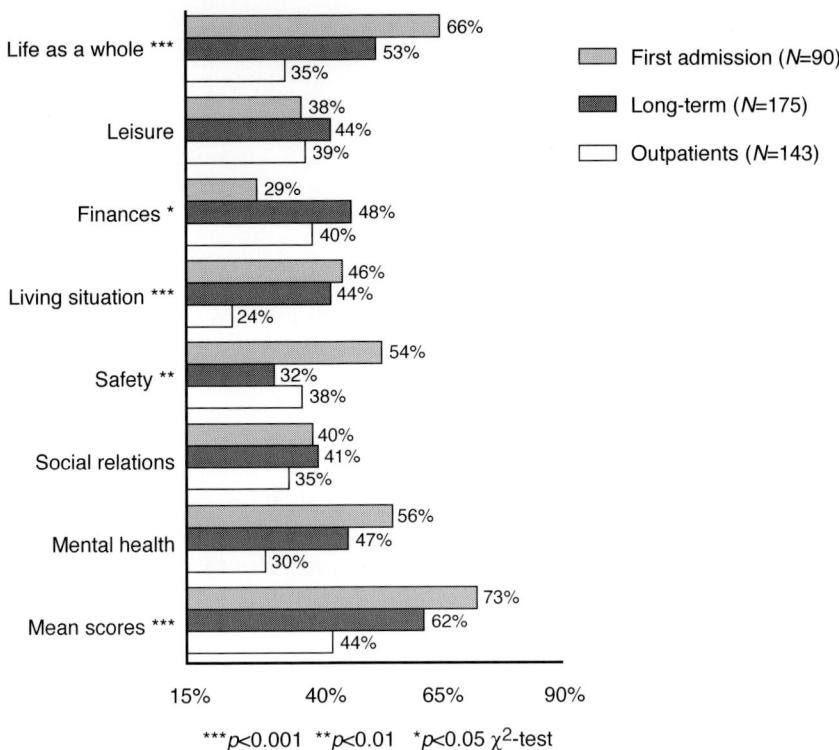

Figure 2. Percentage of patients not satisfied in three samples of patients with schizophrenia.

results are somewhat different. Differences in satisfaction with living situation ($p < 0.01$), safety ($p < 0.001$), life as a whole, and mental health (each $p < 0.05$) remain significant, but the latter two disappear after Bonferroni adjustment. Thus, after controlling for the influence of age and psychopathology, statistically significant differences in satisfaction with only two life domains are left.

This example of data reporting and of statistical analysis may demonstrate that one can safely report dichotomized data and make the results more immediately intelligible to a clinical audience without losing important information. To control for the influence of other factors, however, statistical procedures using the full variance of scores must be applied and, in samples of patients with schizophrenia, age and psychopatholgy are important variables to be regularly controlled for.

Standardization of ratings, data reporting and statistical analysis would be extremely helpful for comparing and utilizing results. Standardized methods must comply with the state of the art in research. Yet, in reporting their results, researchers should keep in mind the interests and needs of clinicians and other groups – including patients – who would like to understand the findings and to draw practical conclusions.

New methods for assessment

New scales to assess patients' subjective quality of life should be appropriate for their purpose. There may be several different purposes, two of which are service evaluation in research and use in clinical practice. Research findings obtained using the existing scales indicate that there are some lessons to be learned for the construction of new scales. One of them is that in previous studies only a few items have been shown to discriminate between settings or to demonstrate change over time. Other data and information may appear interesting, but have no relevance for service evaluation according to empirical evidence. In the light of these findings, the Manchester Short Assessment of Quality of Life (MANSA) has been developed. The MANSA is presented at the end of this book. Application of the MANSA, particularly in repeat interviews, usually does not take more than five minutes. Results have been found to have high concordance with results of the much longer Lancashire Quality of Life Profile on which it is based (Priebe *et al.*, 1999b).

Satisfaction ratings for single life domains have been shown to have little stability over time. Sumscores, however, have been demonstrated to have sufficient stability to be used for examining changes over time that might be due to specific interventions (Kaiser and Priebe, 1998). Thus, sumscores should be used for evaluation, unless there is a specific *a priori* stated hypothesis. Satisfaction ratings with single life domains are to be used only for (i) forming the sumscore, (ii) testing a specific hypothesis, and (iii) generating a specific hypothesis in case the sumscore has shown a significant result.

There are several unanswered questions concerning the use of data yielded by the MANSA, which may be addressed in future studies, e.g. how should the interview situation be standardized to minimize interviewer effects, or which other variables should be routinely controlled for and considered? More data from the general population and from various well-defined patient groups are needed for comparison and for deciding which scores may be regarded as a satisfactory outcome. Obviously, quality of life should be as high as possible, but what is possible to achieve in a given sample and what are reasonable expectations? As Hoffman points out, patients in a given service will hardly improve all the time until they uniformly rate the positive extreme on all rating scales. So, realistic and useful objectives have to be set on the basis of empirical evidence. Information on which scores and which distributions to expect in which population groups, would be helpful for interpreting quality of life data in mentally ill groups. In obtaining data for comparison, as many relevant sociodemographic variables as possible should be controlled for. Such research cannot be undertaken by psychiatrists alone. It needs wider epidemiological and public health studies.

So-called objective variables in quality of life assessment also require serious consideration and specific research. These data, assessed in most quality of life scales, are either trivial or too differentiated to be of great use for evaluation. The influence of very basic objective variables on subjective ratings has been demonstrated, e.g. homelessness (Lehman *et al.*, 1995a) and unemployment (Priebe *et al.*, 1998b) have been shown to be associated with lower subjective quality of life in mentally ill patients. More detailed and specific objective constellations and their association with quality of life scores are, however, difficult to investigate using most of the current scales. Some of the questions, which are used in instruments for assessing objective quality of life indicators in psychiatric patients, were developed decades ago and validated in the general population. It is possible that one might have to start again, developing adequate scales and methods for assessment. This would necessitate empirically based epidemiological and sociological information on which variables distinguish between defined groups in the general population and in patient groups, and which parameters assess relevant social burdens and specific social constellations. For example, most scales assess whether a patient is living with a parent, a partner and children. These three variables are usually analysed separately with no specific underlying hypothesis. Each situation on its own may not present a special burden, while there are special constellations such as that of woman with a job, living with children and parents in the same household, which are particularly burdensome and important to consider in research. This is not likely to be achieved by just developing another scale, but possibly by establishing an ongoing collaboration with epidemiologists and sociologists which would facilitate the use of epidemiological data and sociological and psychological theories in psychiatric quality of life research.

Scores as produced by the MANSA or other scales do not provide detailed information for specific action. If quality of life indicators are to have direct implications for decisions in clinical practice, they should be complemented by qualitative information explaining and specifying patients' quantitative ratings. A new semi-structured or fully structured interview should be developed to assess qualitative information, which is relevant for clinical action. There are three different purposes to be considered in the development of that interview: (i) the interview is to provide clinically useful information on a group level as well as in individual cases, (ii) administering the interview should promote a better relationship between professional carer and patient, and (iii) the interview should also be a training tool directing the interviewer's attention to all relevant aspects in the patient's life; moreover, the interview should be brief to be practicable. Moreover, new ways have to be found for documenting and analysing patients' open answers to standardized questions. The analysis would consider contents and reflect often very specific answers. To conduct the content analysis, better software programmes for routine analysis and presentation of the results in a clear and understandable way should to be developed and made available.

If effects of different mental health services are investigated in controlled or naturalistic long-term studies, the given mental health care system, the characteristics of the services, and all components of treatment that are actually administered should be described exactly. This demand is in response to a shortcoming of evaluative research in general, which also applies to research using the quality of life concept. If a particular service has little or no effect on patients' quality of life, this cannot be interpreted without knowing which mental health care system the patients were treated in and what exactly was done in treatment. Methods to assess all those characteristics in a systematic, valid and useful way are still to be developed (Burns and Priebe, 1996).

Experimental research

In psychology, and to some extent in sociology, there is a fairly long tradition of empirical and experimental research in satisfaction and subjective well-being. In psychiatry, research in quality of life has been more pragmatic and, so far, has had little connection with fundamental psychological research. There are several questions which are difficult to answer without the findings from experimental psychological studies. In which way and to what extent can situational factors influence ratings of patients with different illnesses, e.g. in psychotic and depressed samples? To answer this question, naturalistic studies are insufficient and an experimental design is warranted. The design would involve controlled variation of situational and psychological factors. Of course, there are ethical considerations and various practical problems, which will make such studies difficult to carry out. The author's own experiences with the feasibility of experimental study designs in research with severely mentally ill people are far from encouraging in this respect. One important situational factor of the interview situation, the patient–interviewer relationship, may be systematically altered to assess the influence on ratings. Kaiser *et al.* (1998a) have shown that patients in sheltered accommodation expressed a significantly higher satisfaction with their living situation when they were interviewed by their professional carers than when the interviewer was independent and when confidentiality of ratings was guaranteed. In that study, patients were materially dependent on their keyworkers. In subsequent studies with a similar design in which patients were less dependent on their keyworkers the findings were less conclusive. The influence of the patient–interviewer relationship is very relevant in practical terms. If interviews are done for routine evaluation, an entirely independent interviewer who is in no way involved in care and can assure confidentiality is not a realistic perspective; results about which professional carers are not informed can hardly be used to improve individual care (see Hoffman's chapter). Thus, in most cases, interviewers cannot assure confidentiality concerning patients' statements, and are likely to be involved in the service one way or another. The kind of relationship between patient and interviewer and the degree of dependence within this relationship may vary and influence the results in very different ways. This influence should be assessed in experimental studies and considered in interpretation. On a broader level, experimental studies may help to identify specific emotional and cognitive processes influencing quality of life ratings in different groups and, thus, clarify the concept further.

Experimental designs would also be pertinent in relation to quality of life studies of the immediate effects of neuroleptics, and also of lithium, carbamazepine, benzodiazepines, and other relevant drugs. In randomized controlled clinical trials, long-term effects of different drugs should be examined, which is already the case in most trials testing new antipsychotics. Again, while researchers usually focus on conventional and atypical neuroleptics, the possible impact of other drugs and of psychotherapeutic interventions on quality of life should not be overlooked. The systematic assessment of additional social and psychological variables in such studies allows us to examine whether treatment components that influence quality of life might be mediated further by factors such as frequency of hospitalizations, changes in social situation, or special cognitive coping strategies. For assessing other long-term effects on quality of life ratings, naturalistic studies are needed which would document the influence of street drugs, major life events (including life events associated with treatment such as voluntary or compulsory admission) and living conditions such as homelessness or living alone versus accommodation and/or a partner.

Use of quality of life indicators in the therapeutic process

In short-term studies, but especially in long-term research, quality of life may be considered not only as an evaluation criterion, but also as a factor potentially predicting or influencing outcome. Postrado and Lehman (1995) demonstrated that aspects of quality of life may predict rehospitalizations, and Rudolf and Priebe (1999) found that subgroups of hospitalized patients with alcoholism, identified by patterns of quality of life scores, significantly differed in risk for relapse. Such findings contribute to our understanding of what a positive – or negative – quality of life means for the course of the illness and, subsequently, for the patient's life in the future. Such knowledge is needed if treatment decisions are to be based on quality of life data (Röder-Wanner and Priebe, 1998). The findings reported by Rudolf and Priebe (1999) also indicate that quality of life scores may not only be analysed on the level of whole samples, but may also be used to differentiate between subgroups in a meaningful way and lead to specific interventions, eventually improving outcome.

Quality of life indicators can be used in the individual therapeutic process. Figure 3 displays satisfaction ratings on the Berliner Lebensqualitätsprofil of a 32-year-old patient at two points in time. The first interview was done after the patient was discharged from long-term hospitalization to a sheltered accommodation programme in the community, which is a protected group living arrangement in Berlin. The second interview was conducted 6 months later. In the meantime, the patient had been without a psychotic relapse and without rehospitalization. She had settled in the accommodation scheme and even begun to work. It was a part-time cleaning job, which she coped with successfully. The salary significantly improved her financial situation. So, how did her satisfaction ratings change over the 6-month period?

The patient was more satisfied with her employment situation, which is hardly surprising. She was also more satisfied with her leisure activities, and it may be assumed that this was related to having more money to spend on leisure. She was, however, less satisfied with her financial situation, although she had more money in objective terms. She explained that she was fully aware that she had had less money at the time of the first interview, that was when she was without a job, and for someone who did not work a small amount of money had been acceptable. Now, she did have a job, and for someone who went to work every day she regarded the salary as pretty lousy and was dissatisfied with that situation. Thus, a seemingly contradictory result – more money and less satisfaction – made perfect sense in that individual case when the whole biographical situation was considered. She was also less satisfied with the prospect of staying in the supported accommodation for long – her rating changed from the optimum 7 to a 6. Clinicians regarded that change, although negative in numerical terms, as a positive sign of an increased motivation for moving on from the accommodation scheme to a more independent form of living at a later point of time. There was no change in any other life domain, a result which might have been expected since there was no specific intervention in any other life domain. In a mere analysis of mean scores on a group level, the individual background for the ratings and the consideration of the special circumstances is lost. In most analyses, the ratings of the above patient would contribute to a low association of objective and subjective indicators – positive objective and negative subjective change regarding financial situation – and possibly even to a

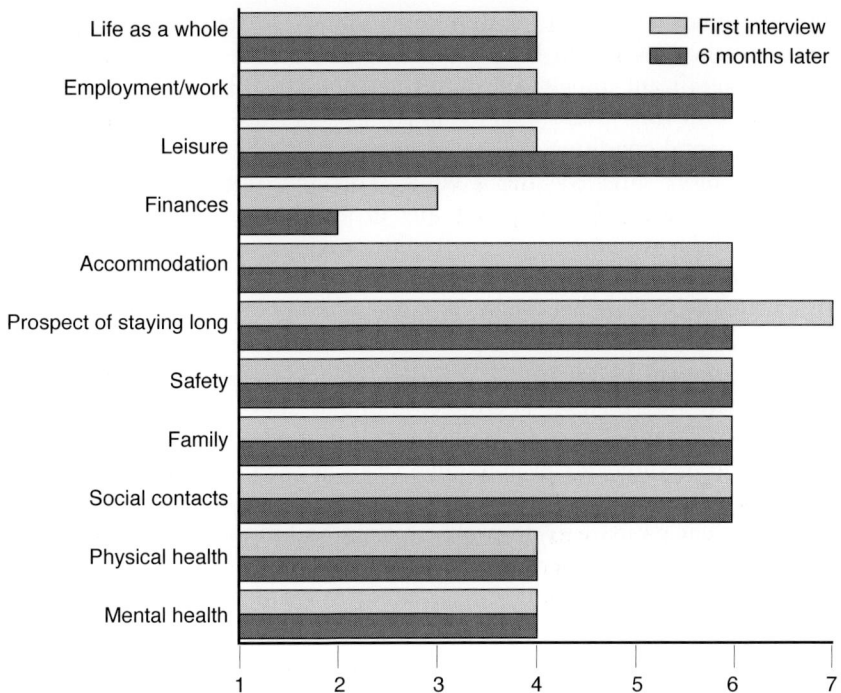

Figure 3. Satisfaction ratings of a patient after admission to a supported accommodation scheme and 6 months later.

unfavourable evaluation of the accommodation scheme, because satisfaction with the prospect of a long-term stay there decreased. The example shows how deceptive results based on mean scores of groups may be. It also indicates that quality of life ratings may be used as a starting point to understand patients' perception and appraisal of life circumstances. A result like the one cited above can form the basis for an intensive talk between the patient and whoever is in charge of treatment to reflect on expectations and achievements. In future intervention studies, quality of life ratings may be regularly assessed and fed back into the therapeutic process. In line with a systematic outcome management, the ratings may be used for modifying treatment decisions. Moreover, specific interventions may be designed and applied for improving quality of life ratings. These interventions might comprise practical support and problem-solving skills training in the case of objectively adverse living situations, and cognitive therapy in the case of what seems an inadequate subjective appraisal of objectively acceptable circumstances. Prospective clinical trials are required to test the effectiveness of such interventions.

For developing cognitive therapy approaches a better understanding of adaptation processes would be helpful. Why do patients with severe mental illness and significant impairment nevertheless frequently show a fairly high satisfaction with their lives? It is assumed that they are able to adjust to an unpleasant mental condition and to an unfavourable life situation over time, and become more satisfied after a while. This adjustment process could be the subject of special research. Mentally ill people seem to have a surprisingly great ability to cope with symptoms, stigma, and adverse life conditions so that in the end they make the best of a difficult situation and are more satisfied with their lives than clinicians often expect. What is this astonishing capability due to, which cognitive processes contribute to it, and how may it be promoted and supported? In the long term, quality of life research might pave the way for new cognitive treatment approaches.

If quality of life indicators are incorporated into outcome management and become useful to clinicians in individual cases, new potentials for evaluation research would be created. Clinicians who are interested in the data are likely to motivate their patients to do proper ratings and to document the findings correctly. This would improve the quality of routinely assessed outcome data so that they can also be used for research. Evaluation could be based on widely available, reliable and valid routine data, and not primarily on findings of specific studies in model institutions, which are difficult to generalize.

Appendix

The Manchester Short Assessment of Quality of Life (MANSA)

STEFAN PRIEBE, PETER HUXLEY, SUSAN KNIGHT and SHERRILL EVANS

Section 1

Date of birth		□□ □□ □□
Gender	1=Male, 2=Female	□
Ethnic origin	1=White, 2=Black Caribbean, 3=Black African, 4=Black other, 5=Indian, 6=Pakistani, 7=Bangladeshi, 8=Chinese, 9=Other	□
Diagnosis	Use ICD 10, DSM-IV or any other coding system that is in place in your service	

Section 2

In a first interview, ask all questions 1 to 9. In a repeat interview, ask first, whether there have been any changes in the respondent's circumstances as assessed in Section 2. If the answer is yes, complete questions 1 to 9. If the answer is no, go straight to Section 3 (question 10).

1 Age at leaving full time education □□

2 Employment status 1=In paid employment, 2=In sheltered employment, 3=Training/education is main occupation, 4=Unemployed, 5=Retired, 6=Other □

If employed, ask questions 3 and 4, otherwise go straight to question 5

3 What is your occupation? ....

4 How many hours a week do you work? □□

5 What is your total monthly income after tax? □□□□

6 Which if any state benefits do you receive? ....

7 How many children (if any) do you have? □□

8 Who else (if anybody) do you live with? 1=Live alone, 2=With partner, 3=With parents, 4=With child/children under 18, 5=With child/children over 18, 6=Other (please specify) □

9 In which type of residence do you currently live?
                        01=House/flat (owner occupied),
                        02=House/flat (Housing association)
                        03=House/flat (private rent), 04=Boarding out
                        (incl B+B)
                        05=Hostel, supported/group home,
                        06=Sheltered housing,
                        07=Residential home, 09=Hospital ward,
                        10=No fixed abode   □□

Section 3

All questions in this section are to be asked every time the
instrument is applied.
10 How satisfied are you with your life as a whole today?*   □
11 How satisfied are you with your job (or sheltered employ-
    ment, or training/education as your main occupation)?*   □
    or if unemployed or retired
    How satisfied are you with being unemployed/retired?*   □
12 How satisfied are you with your financial situation?*   □
13 Do you have anyone who you would call a 'close friend'?
    1=Yes, 2=No   □
14 In the last week have you seen a friend (visited a friend,
    been visited by a friend, or met a friend outside both your
    home and work)?
    1=Yes, 2=No   □
15 How satisfied are you with the number and quality of your
    friendships?*   □
16 How satisfied are you with your leisure activities?*   □
17 How satisfied are you with your accommodation?*   □
18 In the past year have you been accused of a crime?
    1=Yes, 2=No   □
19 In the past year have you been a victim of physical violence?
    1=Yes, 2=No   □
20 How satisfied are you with your personal safety?*   □
21 How satisfied are you with the people that you live with?*   □
    or if you live alone
    How satisfied are you with living alone?*   □
22 How satisfied are you with your sex life?*   □
23 How satisfied are you with your relationship with your
    family?*   □
24 How satisfied are you with your physical health?*   □
25 How satisfied are you with your mental health?*   □

*Use the Satisfaction Scale below

Satisfaction Scale

1	2	3	4	5	6	7
Couldn't be worse	Displeased	Mostly dissatisfied	Mixed	Mostly satisfied	Pleased	Couldn't be better

Specific instructions

ID

It is important to be able to identify the respondent, to ensure that respondent's details are not included in any analysis more than once. Please affix the respondent's name, address and a Client Identification number.

Section 2

2.   Only respondents who receive an income commensurate with the hours worked should be classed as being in paid employment. Those engaged in work experience, work training or education while receiving unemployment benefit should be classed as unemployed.

6.   If the respondent shares an income with a partner, the answer to this question should be calculated by adding these incomes together and then dividing by two.

8.   Where a respondent lives with children aged under 18 and over 18, under 18s take precedence and code 4 should be entered in the box.

Section 3

The satisfaction questions should be answered using the Satisfaction Scale. The respondent can be given a card showing the Satisfaction Scale at the beginning of the interview, for them to keep for the duration of the interview. The Satisfaction Scale is numbered from 1 (low) to 7 (high); the number corresponding to the respondent's answer should be recorded in the appropriate box for each 'satisfaction' question.

18.   In situations where a respondent has no 'close friend' but indicates that they consider a family member to be a 'close friend' this should be included as an appropriate response. However, if in these circumstances the respondent cites a professional as a 'close friend' this should not be considered appropriate.

20.   This question relates to those other family members who do not live with the respondent.

22.   This question should be asked of all respondents, whether or not they have an active sex life. In the latter case it relates to their satisfaction with not having an active sex life.

References

Aaronson, N.K. (1989). Quality of life assessment in clinical trials: methodological issues. *Controlled Clinical Trials*, **10**, 195–208.

Aaronson, N.K. (1993). The EORTC QLQ-C30: a quality of life instrument for use in international clinical trials in oncology. *Quality of Life Research*, **2**, 51.

Abbey, A. and Andrews, F.M. (1985). Modelling the psychological determinants of life quality. *Social Indicators Research*, **16**, 1–34.

Abele, A. and Becker, P. (1991). *Wohlbefinden Theorie Empirie Diagnostik*. Juventa, Weinheim und München.

Aberg-Wistedt, A., Cressell, T., Lidberg, Y., Liljenberg, B. and Ösby, U. (1995). Two year outcome of team-based intensive case management for patients with schizophrenia. *Psychiatric Services*, **46**, 1263–1266.

Ager, A. (1990). *Life Experiences Checklist*. NFER Nelson, Windsor.

Ajzen, I. and Fishbein, M. (1980). *Understanding Attitudes and Predicting Social Behaviour*. Prentice Hall, Englewood Cliffs.

American Psychiatric Association (1980). *Diagnostic and Statistical Manual of Mental Disorders – Third Edition*. APA, Washington DC.

Andrews, F.M. (Ed.) (1986). *Research on the Quality of Life*. University of Michigan, Institute for Social Research, Ann Arbor.

Andrews, F.M. and Withey, S.B. (1974). Developing measures of perceived quality of life: results from several national surveys. *Social Indicators Research* **1**, 1–26.

Andrews, F.M. and Withey, S.B. (1976). *Social Indicators of Well-being: Americans' Perceptions of Life Quality*. Plenum Press, New York.

Angermeyer, M.C. (1994). Symptomfreiheit oder Lebensqualität: Ziele der Schizophreniebehandlung. In: Katschnig, H. and König, P. (Eds), *Schizophrenie und Lebensqualität*. Springer, Vienna, pp. 65–80.

Angermeyer, M.C. and Katschnig, H. (1997). Psychotropic medication and quality of life: a conceptual framework for assessing their relationship. In: Katschnig, H., Freeman, H. and Sartorius, N. (Eds), *Quality of Life in Mental Disorders*. Wiley, Chichester, pp. 215–225.

Angermeyer, M.C. and Kilian, R. (1997). Theoretical models of quality of life for mental disorders. In: Katschnig, H., Freeman, H. and Sartorius, N. (Eds). *Quality of Life in Mental Disorders*. Wiley, Chichester, pp. 19–30.

Angst, J., Bech, P., Engel, R. *et al.* (1991). Report on the third consensus conference on the methodology of clinical trials with antipsychotic drugs. *Pharmacopsychiatry*, **24**, 149–152.

Angst, J., Bech, P., Bruinvels, J. *et al.* (1994). Report on the fifth consensus conference: methodology of long-term clinical trials in psychiatry. *Pharmacopsychiatry*, **27**, 101–107.

Anthony, W.A., Cohen, M.R. and Vitalo, R. (1978). The measurement of rehabilitation outcome. *Schizophrenia Bulletin*, **4**, 365–383.

Arns, P.G. and Linney, J.A. (1993). Work, self and life satisfaction for persons with severe and persistent mental disorders. *Psychosocial Rehabilitation Journal*, 17, 63–79.

Atkinson, J.A., Coia, D.A., Gilmour, W.H. and Harper, J.P. (1996). The impact of education groups for people with schizophrenia on social functioning and quality of life. *British Journal of Psychiatry*, 168, 199–204.

Atkinson, M., Zibin, S. and Chuang, H. (1997). Characterising quality of life among patients with chronic mental illness: a critical examination of self-report methodology. *American Journal of Psychiatry*, 154, 99–105.

Audit Commission (1994). *Finding a Place: A Review of Mental Health Services for Adults*. HMSO, London.

Avison, W.R. and Speechley, K.N. (1987). The discharged psychiatric patient: a review of social, social–psychological, and psychiatric correlates of outcome. *American Journal of Psychiatry*, 144, 10–18.

Awad, A.G. (1992). Quality of life of schizophrenic patients on medications and implications for new drug trials. *Hospital and Community Psychiatry*, 2, 262–265.

Awad, A.G. (1993). Subjective response to neuroleptics in schizophrenia. *Schizophrenia Bulletin*, 19, 609–618.

Awad, A.G. (1995). Quality of life issues in medicated schizophrenics: therapeutic and research implications. In: Shriqui, C. and Nasrallah, H. (Eds). *Contemporary Issues in the Treatment of Schizophrenia*. American Psychiatric Press, Washington, pp. 735–747.

Awad, A.G. and Hogan, T.P. (1994). Subjective response to neuroleptics and the quality of life: implications for treatment outcome. *Acta Psychiatrica Scandinavica*, 89 (Suppl. 380), 27–32.

Awad, A.G., Hogan, T.P., Voruganti, L.N.P. and Heslegrave, R.J. (1995a). Patients' subjective experiences on antipsychotic medications: implications for outcome and quality of life. *International Clinical Psychopharmacology*, 10 (Suppl. 3), 123–133.

Awad, A.G., Voruganti, L.N.P. and Heslegrave, R.J. (1995b). The aims of anti-psychotic medications: what are they and are they being achieved? *CNS Drugs*, 4, 8–16.

Awad, A.G., Lapierre, Y., Angus, C. and Rylander, A. (1997a). Quality of life and response of negative symptoms in schizophrenia to haloperidol and the atypical antipsychotic remoxipride. *Journal of Psychiatry and Neuroscience*, 22, 244–248.

Awad, A.G., Voruganti, L.N.P. and Heslegrave, R.J. (1997b). A conceptual model of quality of life in schizophrenia: description and preliminary validation. *Quality of Life Research*, 6, 21–26.

Awad, A.G., Voruganti, L.N.P. and Heslegrave, R.J. (1997c). Measuring quality of life in patients with schizophrenia. *PharmacoEconomics*, 11, 32–47.

Bagne, C.A. and Lewis, R.F. (1992). Evaluating the effects of drugs on behaviour and quality of life: an alternative strategy for clinical trials. *Journal of Consulting and Clinical Psychology*, 60, 225–239.

Baker, R. and Hall, J. (1983). *Users Manual for Rehabilitation Evaluation*. Hall and Baker, Aberdeen.

Baker, F. and Intagliata, J. (1982). Quality of life in the evaluation of community support systems. *Evaluation and Program Planning*, 5, 69–79.

Baker, F., Jodrey, D. and Intagliata, J. (1992). Social support and quality of life of community support clients. *Community Mental Health Journal*, 28, 397–411.

Baldwin, S. (1986). Problems with needs where theory meets practice. *Disability, Handicap and Society*, 1, 139–145.

Baldwin, S., Baser, C. and Harding, K. (1999). *Multilevel Needs Assessment*. BABP, London, in press.

Barnes, T.R.E. (1989). A rating scale for drug-induced akathisia. *British Journal of Psychiatry*, 154, 672–676.

Barrowclough, C. and Fleming, I. (1986). *Goal Planning with Elderly People*. Manchester University Press, Manchester.

Barry, M.M. (1997). Well-being and life satisfaction as components of quality of life in mental disorders. In: Katschnig, H., Freeman, H. and Sartorius, N. (Eds), *Quality of Life in Mental Disorders*, Wiley, Chichester, pp. 31–42.

Barry, M.M. and Crosby, C. (1996). Quality of life as an evaluative measure in assessing the impact of community care on people with long-term psychiatric disorders. *British Journal of Psychiatry*, **168**, 210–216.

Barry, M.M. and Zissi, A. (1997). Quality of life as an outcome measure in evaluating mental health services: a review of the empirical evidence. *Social Psychiatry Epidemiology*, **32**, 38–47.

Barry, M.M., Crosby, C. and Boog, J. (1993). Methodological issues in evaluating the quality of life of long stay psychiatric patients. *Journal of Mental Health*, **2**, 43–56.

Baumann, U., Fähndrich, E., Stieglitz, R.D. and Woggon, B. (Eds) (1990). *Measurement of Change in Psychiatry and Clinical Psychology*. Profil, Munich.

Beck, A.T., Ward, C., Mendelson, M., Mock, J. and Erbaugh, J. (1961). An inventory for measuring depression. *Archives of General Psychiatry*, **4**, 561–571.

Becker, T. (1995). Die Schließung psychiatrischer Großkrankenhäuser in England: Evaluation durch das TAPS-Projekt -Ein Literaturbericht. *Psychiatrische Praxis*, **22**, 50–54.

Becker, M., Diamond, R. and Sainfort, F. (1993). A new patient focused index for measuring quality of life in persons with severe and persistent mental illness. *Quality of Life Research*, **2**, 239–251.

Bergner, M., Bobbitt, R.A., Kressel, S., Pollard, W.E., Gilson, B.S. and Morris, J.R. (1976). The Sickness Impact Profile: conceptual formulation and methodology for the development of a health status measure. *International Journal Health Services*, **6**, 393–415.

Bergner, M., Bobbit, R.A., Carter, W.B. and Gilson, B.S. (1981). The Sickness Impact Profile: development and final revision of a health status measure. *Medical Care*, **19**, 787–805.

Bigelow, D.A. and Young, D.J. (1991). Effectiveness of a case management program. *Community Mental Health Journal*, **27**, 115–123.

Bigelow, D.A., Brodsky, G., Stewart, L. and Olson, M. (1982). The concept and measurement of quality of life as a dependent variable in evaluation of mental health services. In: Stahler, G.J. and Tash, W.R. (Eds), *Innovative Approaches to Mental Health Evaluation*. Academic Press, New York, pp. 345–366.

Bigelow, D.A., Gareau, M.J. and Young, D.J. (1990). A quality of life interview. *Psychosocial Rehabilitation Journal*, **14**, 94–98.

Bigelow, D.A., McFarland, B.H. and Olson, M.M. (1991). Quality of life of community mental health programme clients: validating a measure. *Community Mental Health Journal*, **27**, 43–55.

Blyler, C.R. and Fenton, W.S. (1997). Satisfaction with treatment outcome and non-compliance in schizophrenia. *Schizophrenia Research*, **24**, 201–205.

Bond, G.R., Miller, L.D., Krumwied, R.D. and Ward, R.S. (1988). Assertive case management in three CMHCs: a controlled study. *Hospital and Community Psychiatry*, **39**, 411–418.

Bond, G.R., Witheridge, T.F., Wasmer, D., Dincin, J., McRae, S.A., Mayes, J. and Ward, R.S. (1989). A comparison of two crises housing alternatives to psychiatric hospitalisation. *Hospital and Community Psychiatry*, **40**, 177–183.

Bond, G.R., Witheridge, T.F., Dincin, J., Wasmer, D., Webb, J. and de Graaf-Kaser, R. (1990). Assertive community treatment for frequent users of psychiatric hospitals in a large city: a controlled study. *American Journal of Community Psychology*, **18**, 865–891.

Bond, G.R., McDonel, E.C., Miller, L.D. and Pensec, M. (1991). Assertive community treatment and reference groups: an evaluation of their effectiveness for young adults with serious mental illness and substance abuse problems. *Psychosocial Rehabilitation Journal*, **15**, 31–43.

Borland, A., McRae, J. and Lycan, C. (1989). Outcomes of five years of continuous intensive case management. *Hospital and Community Psychiatry*, 40, 369–376.

Bowling, A. (1991). *Measuring Health: A Review of Quality of Life*. Open University Press, Milton Keynes.

Bowling, A. (1995). *Measuring Disease. A Review of Disease-Specific Quality of Life Measurements*. Open University Press, Milton Keynes.

Bradburn, N.M. (1965). *Affect Balance Scale*. Aldine, Chicago.

Bradburn, N.M. (1969). *The Structure of Psychological Well-Being*. Aldine, Chicago.

Brenner (1973). *Mental Illness and The Economy*. Harvard University Press, Cambridge, MA.

Brewin, C.R. (1992). Measuring individual needs for care and services. In: Thornicroft, G., Brewin, C.R. and Wing, J. (Eds), *Measuring Mental Health Needs*. Gaskell, London.

Brickman, P., Coates, D. and Janoff-Bulman, R. (1978). Lottery winners and accident victims: is happiness relative? *Journal of Personality and Social Psychology* 36, 917–927.

Bridges, K., Huxley, P. and Oliver, J. (1994). Psychiatric rehabilitation: redefined for the 1990s. *International Journal of Social Psychiatry*, 40, 1–16.

Bröker, M., Rohricht, F. and Priebe, S. (1965). Initial assessment of hospital treatment by patients with paranoid schizophrenia: a predictor of outcome. *Psychiatry Research*, 58, 77–81.

Brown, I., Renwick, R. and Nagler, M. (1996). The centrality of quality of life in health promotion and rehabilitation. In: Renwick, R., Brown, I. and Nagler, M. (Eds), *Quality of Life in Health Promotion and Rehabilitation. Conceptual Approaches, Issues, and Applications*. Russell Sage Foundation, Thousand Oaks, pp. 3–13.

Browne, S., Roe, M., Lane, A., Gervin, M., Morris, M., Kinsella, A., Larkin, C. and O'Callaghan, E. (1996). A preliminary report on the effect of a psychosocial and educative programme on quality of life and symptomatology in schizophrenia. *European Psychiatry*, 11, 386–389.

Browne, S., Garavan, J., Gervin, M., Roe, M., Larkin, C. and O'Callaghan, E. (1998). Quality of life. In: Schizophrenia: Insight and Subjective Response to Neuroleptics. *Journal of Nervous and Mental Disease*, 186, 74–78.

Bullinger, M., (1991). Erhebungsmethoden. In: Tüchler, H. and Lutz, D. (Eds), *Lebensqualität und Krankheit. Auf dem Weg zu einem medizinischen Kriterium Lebensqualität*. Deutscher Ärzte-Verlag, Cologne, pp. 85–96.

Bullinger, M., Anderson, R., Cella, D. and Aaronson, N. (1993). Developing and evaluating cross-cultural instruments from minimum requirements to optimal models. *Quality of Life Research*, 2, 451–459.

Burnham, M.A., Wells, K.B., Leake, B. and Landsverk, J. (1988). Development of a brief screening instrument for detecting depressive disorders. *Medical Care*, 26, 775–789.

Burns, T. and Priebe, S. (1996). Mental health care systems and their characteristics: a proposal. *Acta Psychiatrica Scandinavica*, 94, 381–385.

Calman, K.C. (1984). Quality of life in cancer patients – a hypothesis. *Journal of Medical Ethics*, 10, 124–127; 1551–1555.

Campbell, A. and Rodgers, W.L. (1972). *The Human Meaning of Social Change*. Russell Sage Foundation, New York.

Campbell, A., Converse, P.E. and Rodgers, W.L. (1976). *The Quality of American Life: Perceptions, Evaluations, and Satisfactions*. Russell Sage Foundation, New York.

Campbell, J., Schraiber, R., Temkin, T. and Ten Tuscher, T. (1989). *The Well-Being Project: Mental Health Clients Speak for Themselves*. Report to the Californian Department of Mental Health.

Caplan, G. (1994). *Principles of Preventive Psychiatry*. Basic Books, New York.

Caron, J., Tempier, R., Mercier, C. and Leouffre, P. (1998). Components of social support and quality of life in severely mentally ill, low income individuals and in general population. *Community Mental Health Journal*, 34, 459–475.

Casey, D.E. (1994). Motor and mental aspects of acute extrapyramidal syndromes. *Acta Psychiatrica Scandinavica*, **89** (Suppl. 380), 14–20.

Champney, T.F. and Dzurec, L.C. (1992). Involvement in productive activities and satisfaction with living situation among severely mentally disabled adults. *Hospital and Community Psychiatry*, **43**, 899–903.

Chandler, D., Meisel, J., McGowen, M., Mintz, J. and Madison, K. (1996). Client outcomes in two model capitated integrated service agencies. *Psychiatric Services*, **47**, 175–180.

Cheng, S.T. (1988). Subjective quality of life in the planning and evaluation of programmes. *Evaluation and Programme Planning*, **11**, 123–134.

Chouinard, G., Ross-Chouinard, A. and Annable, L. (1980). The extrapyramidal symptom rating scale. *Canadian Journal of Neurological Sciences*, **7**, 233.

Clare, A.W. and Cairns, V.E. (1979). Design, development and use of a standardised interview to assess social maladjustment and dysfunction in community samples. *Psychological Medicine*, **8**, 589–604.

Cohen, J. (1988). *Statistical Power Analysis for the Behavioural Sciences*. Erlbaum, Hillsdale.

Coid, J.W. (1993). Quality of life for patients detained in hospital. *British Journal of Psychiatry*, **162**, 611–620.

Corrigan, P.W. and Buican, B. (1995). The construct validity of subjective quality of life for the severely mentally ill. *Journal of Nervous and Mental Disease*, **183**, 281–285.

Corrigan, P.W., Liberman, R.P. and Engle, J.D. (1990). From noncompliance to collaboration in the treatment of schizophrenia. *Hospital and Community Psychiatry*, **41**, 1203–1211.

Corten, P., Mercier, C. and Pelc, I. (1994). Subjective quality of life: clinical model for assessment of rehabilitation in psychiatry. *Social Psychiatry and Psychiatric Epidemiology*, **29**, 178–183.

Cronbach, L.J. (1947). Test 'reliability': its meaning and determination. *Psychometrika*, **12**, 1–16.

Cronbach, L.J. and Meehl, P.E. (1955). Construct validity in psychological test. *Psychological Bulletin*, **52**, 281–302.

Croog, S.H., Levine, S., Testa, M.A. *et al.* (1986). The effects of anti-hypertensive therapy on the quality of life. *The New England Journal of Medicine*, **314**, 1657–1664.

Cullen, D., Waite, A., Oliver, N., Carson, J. and Holloway, F. (1997). Case management for the mentally ill: a comparative evaluation of client satisfaction. *Health and Social Care in the Community*, **5**, 106–115.

Cutler, D.L., Tatum, E. and Shore, J.H. (1987). A comparison of schizophrenic patients in different community support treatment approaches. *Community Mental Health Journal*, **23**, 103–113.

Davies, A. and Huxley, P.J. (1997). Final report on *Modes of Opiate Abuse Treatment in Three Areas* to The NHSE R&D Division. School of Psychiatry, The University of Manchester, Manchester.

Day, H. and Jankey, S.G. (1996). Lessons from the literature: toward a holistic model of quality of life. In: Renwick, R., Brown, I. and Nagler, M. (Eds), *Quality of Life in Health Promotion and Rehabilitation. Conceptual Approaches, Issues, and Applications*. Russell Sage Foundation, Thousand Oaks, pp. 39–50.

De Haes, J.C., Van Ostrom, M.A. and Welvaart, K. (1986). The effect of radical and conserving surgery on the quality of life of early breast cancer patients. *European Journal of Social Oncology*, **12**, 337–342.

Department of Health (1990). *The Care Programme Approach for People with a Mental Illness Referred to the Specialist Psychiatric Services*. Department of Health, London.

Department of Health (1994). *Guidance on the Discharge of Mentally Disordered People and Their Continuing Care in the Community*. Department of Health, London.

Department of Health (1995). *Building Bridges. A Guide To Arrangements For Inter-agency Working For The Care and Protection of Severely Mentally Ill People*. Department of Health, London.

Derogatis, L.R. (1993). *BSI – Brief Symptom Inventory: Administration, Scoring and Procedures Manual*. National Computer Systems, Minneapolis, MN.

Diamond, R. (1985). Drugs and the quality of life: the patient's point of view. *Journal of Clinical Psychiatry*, **46**, 29–35.

Dickerson, F.B. (1997). Assessing clinical outcomes: the community functioning of persons with serious mental illness. *Psychiatric Services*, **48**, 897–902.

Dickerson, F.B., Boronow, J.J., Ringel, N. and Parente, F. (1997). Lack of insight among outpatients with schizophrenia. *Psychiatric Services*, **49**, 195–199.

Diener, E. (1984). Subjective well-being. *Psychological Bulletin*, **95**, 542–575.

Dilling, H., Mombour, W. and Schmidt, M.H. (Eds) (1991). *Internationale Klassifikation Psychischer Störungen – ICD 10*. Huber, Bern.

Dodrill, C.B. (1978). A neuropsychological battery for epilepsy. *Epilepsia*, **19**, 611–623.

Drake, R.E., McHugo, G.J., Becker, D.R., Anthony, W.A. and Clark, R.E. (1996). The New Hampshire study of supported employment for people with severe mental illness. *Journal of Consulting and Clinical Psychology*, **64**, 391–399.

Drake, R.E., Yovetich, N.A., Bebout, R.R., Harris, M. and McHugo, G.J. (1997). Integrated treatment for dually diagnosed homeless adults. *Journal of Nervous and Mental Disease*, **185**, 298–305.

Dunbar, G.C., Stroker, M.J., Hodges, T.C. and Beaumont, G. (1992). The development of the SBQOL: a unique scale for measuring quality of life. *British Journal of Health Economics*, **2**, 65–74.

Dupuy, H.J. (1973). *Developmental Rationale, Substantive, Derivatable, and Conceptual Relevance of the General Well-Being Schedule*. National Centre for Health Statistics, Fairfax, VA.

Earls, M. and Nelson, G. (1988). The relationship between long-term psychiatric clients' psychological well-being and their perceptions of housing and social support. *American Journal of Community Psychology*, **16**, 279–293.

Ebrahim, S. (1995). Clinical and public health perspectives and applications of health-related quality of life measurement. *Social Science and Medicine*, **41**, 1383–1394.

Editorial (1995). Quality of life and clinical trials. *Lancet*, **346**, 1–2.

Emerson, E.B. (1985). Evaluating the impact of deinstitutionalization on the lives of mentally retarded people. *American Journal of Mental Deficiency*, **90**, 277–288.

Endicott, J., Spitzer, R.L., Fleiss, J.L. and Cohen, J. (1976). The Global Assessment Scale: a procedure for measuring overall severity of psychiatric disturbance. *Archives General Psychiatry*, **33**, 766–771.

Evans, S. (1998). Self-report Methodology in QOL Measurement. Paper presented at the 12th European Health Psychology Conference, Vienna, September 1998.

Fabian, E.S. (1989). Work and the quality of life. *Psychosocial Rehabilitation Journal*, **12**, 39–49.

Fabian, E.S. (1990). Quality of life: a review of theory and practice implications for individuals with long-term mental illness. *Rehabilitation Psychology*, **35**, 161–170.

Farquahar, M. (1995). Definitions of quality of life: a taxonomy. *Journal of Advanced Nursing*, **22**, 502–508.

Feinstein, A.R. (1987). Clinimetric perspectives. *Journal of Chronic Diseases*, **40**, 635–640.

Felce, D. and Perry, L. (1995). Quality of life: its definition and measurement. *Research in Developmental Disabilities*, **16**, 51–74.

Felce, D. and Perry, J. (1996). Exploring current conceptions of quality of life: a model for people with and without disabilities. In: Renwick, R., Brown, I. and Nagler, M. (Eds). *Quality of Life in Health Promotion and Rehabilitation. Conceptual Approaches, Issues, and Applications*. Russell Sage Foundation, Thousand Oaks, pp. 51–62.

Felton, C.J., Stastny, P., Shern, D.L. *et al.* (1995). Consumers as peer specialists on intensive case management teams: impact on client outcomes. *Psychiatric Services*, **46**, 1937–1044.

Ferrans, C.E. and Powers, M.J. (1985). Quality of Life Index: development and psycho-metric properties. *Advances in Nursing Science*, **8**, 15–24.

Fitzpatrick, R. (1994). Applications of health status measures. In: Jenkinson, C. (Ed.). *Measuring Health and Medical Outcomes*. University College London Press, London.

Fitzpatrick, R., Fletcher, A., Gore, S., Jones, D., Spiegelhalter, D. and Cox, D. (1992). Quality of life measures in health care. In: Applications and Issues in Assessment. *British Medical Journal*, 305, 1074–1077.

Franklin, J.L., Simmons, J., Solovitz, B., Clemons, J.R. and Miller, G.E. (1986). Assessing quality of life of the mentally ill: a three-dimensional model. *Evaluation and The Health Professions*, 9, 376–388.

Franklin, J.L., Solovitz, B., Mason, M., Clemons, J.R. and Miller, G.E. (1987). An evaluation of case management. *American Journal of Public Health*, 77, 674–678.

Franz, M., Plüddemann, K., Gruppe, H. and Gallhofer, B. (1996). Modifikation und Anwendung der Münchner Lebensqualitäts-Dimensionen-Liste bei schizophrenen Patienten. In: Möller, H.J., Engel, R.R. and Hoff, P. (Eds), *Befunderhebung in der Psychiatrie: Lebensqualität, Negativsymptomatik und andere aktuelle Entwicklungen*. Springer, Vienna, pp. 103–111.

Franz, M., Lis, S., Pluddemann, K. and Gallhofer, B. (1997). Conventional versus atypical neuroleptics: subjective quality of life in schizophrenic patients. *British Journal of Psychiatry*, 170, 422–425.

Gannon, L., Vaux, A., Rhodes, K. and Luchetta, T. (1992). A two-domain model of well-being: everyday events, social support, and gender-related factors. *Journal of Research in Personality*, 26, 288–301.

Gibbons, J.S. and Butler, J.P. (1987). Quality of life for "new" long-stay psychiatric in-patients: the effects of moving to a hostel. *British Journal of Psychiatry*, 151, 347–354.

Gill, T.M. and Feinstein, A.R. (1994). A critical appraisal of the quality of life measurements. *Journal of the American Medical Association*, 272, 619–626.

Glaser, B.G. and Strauss, A.L. (1967). *The Discovery of Grounded Theory: Strategies for Qualitative Research*. Aldine de Gruyter, New York.

Glatzer, W. (1984). Zufriedenheitsunterschiede zwischen Lebensbereichen. In: Glatzer, W. and Zapf, W. (Eds). *Lebensqualität in der Bundesrepublik*. Campus, Frankfurt.

Glatzer, W. and Zapf, W. (Eds) (1984). *Quality of Life in the Federal Republic of Germany*. Campus, Frankfurt.

Glover, G. (1995). Mental health informatics and the rhythm of community care. *British Medical Journal*, 311, 1038–1039.

Glover, G. and Oliver, J.P.J. (1999). How are you doing with your mental health care? *Nursing Times*, in press.

Goldberg, D.P. (1972). *The Detection of Psychiatric Illness by Questionnaire*, Maudsley Monograph No. 21, Oxford University Press, Oxford.

Goldman, H.H., Skodol, A.E. and Lave, T.R. (1992). Revising axis V for DSM-IV: a review of measures of social functioning. *American Journal of Psychiatry*, 149, 1148–1156.

Gotay, C.C., Korn, E.L., McCabe, J.S., Moore, T.D. and Cheson, B.D. (1992). Quality of life assessment in cancer treatment protocols: research issues in protocol development. *Journal of the National Cancer Institute*, 84, 575–579.

Gurland, B.J., Yorkston, N.J., Stone, A.R. and Frank, J.D. (1972). The structured and scaled interview to assess maladjustment (SSIAM): description, rationale and development. *Archives of General Psychiatry*, 27, 259–264.

Guy, W. (1976). *ECDEU Assessment Manual for Psychopharmacology*. Department of Health, Education and Welfare, Washington DC.

Guyatt, G.H. and Jaeschke, R. (1990). Measurements in clinical trials: choosing the appropriate approach. In: Spilker, B. (Ed.), *Quality of Life Assessments in Clinical Trials*. Raven, New York, pp. 37–46.

Guyatt, G.H., Bombardier, C. and Tugwell, P.X. (1986). Measuring disease-specific quality of life in clinical trials. *Canadian Medical Association Journal*, 134, 889–895.

Guyatt, G.H., Veldhuyzen van Zanten, S.J.O., Feeny, D.H. and Patrick, D.L. (1989). Measuring quality of life in clinical trials: a taxonomy and review. *Canadian Medical Association Journal*, 140, 1441–1448.

Hachey, R. and Mercier, C. (1993). The impact of rehabilitation services on the quality of life of chronic mental patients. *Occupational Therapy in Mental Health*, 12, 1–26.

Handal, P.J. and Moore, C. (1987). The influence of physical, psychosocial, and socio-cultural supplies on mental health and life satisfaction: a test of Caplan's supply model. *Journal of Primary Prevention*, 7, 132–142.

Hansson, L. (1996). Sectorized services outcome research. In: Knudsen, H.C. and Thornicroft, G. (Eds), *Mental Health Service Evaluation*. Cambridge University Press, Cambridge.

Hansson, L. and Höglund, E. (1995). Patient satisfaction with psychiatric services. The development, reliability and validity of two patient satisfaction questionnaires for use in in-patient and outpatient settings. *Nordic Journal of Psychiatry*, 49, 257–262.

Harris, M. (1968). *The Rise of Anthropological Theory: A History of Theories of Culture.* Thomas Y. Crowell, New York.

Harris, M. (1979). *Cultural Materialism: The Struggle for a Science of Culture.* Random House, New York.

Heinrichs, D.W., Hanlon, T.E. and Carpenter, W.T. (1984). The Quality of Life Scale: an instrument for rating the schizophrenia deficit syndrome. *Schizophrenia Bulletin*, 10, 388–398.

Heinze, M. and Priebe, S. (1995). On the term needs in psychiatric research (in German). *Fundamenta Psychiatrica*, 9, 52–60.

Heinze, M., Taylor, R., Priebe, S. and Thornicroft, G. (1997). The quality of life of patients with paranoid schizophrenia in London and Berlin. *Social Psychiatry and Psychiatric Epidemiology*, 32, 292–297.

Helmchen, H. (1990). 'Lebensqualität' als Bewertungskriterium in der Psychiatrie. In: Scholmerich, P. and Thews, G. (Eds), *'Lebensqualität' als Bewertungskriterium in der Medizin. Symposium der Akademie der Wissenschaften und der Literatur, Mainz.* Fischer, Stuttgart, pp. 93–115.

Heslegrave, R.J., Awad, A.G. and Voruganti, L.N.P. (1997a). Assessing quality of life in persons with neurocognitive deficits and chronic mental illness: lessons from a non-disability study. *Journal on Developmental Disabilities*, 5, 77–90.

Heslegrave, R.J., Awad, A.G. and Voruganti, L.N.P. (1997b). The influence of neurocognitive deficits and symptoms on quality of life in schizophrenia. *Journal of Psychiatry and Neuroscience*, 22, 235–243.

Heyrman, J. and Van Hoeck, K. (1993). Measuring health outcome: shouldn't we first define health? Paper presented to the WONCA/SIMG Congress on Quality of Care in Family Medicine/General Practice. The Hague, Netherlands, June 13–17 1993.

Hinterhuber, H., Holzner, B., Kemmler, G. *et al.* (1995). Verläufe schizophrener Psychosen. Die Tiroler Langzeitstudie. In: Hinterhuber, H., Fleischhacker, W.W. and Meise, U. (Eds), *Die Behandlung der Schizophrenien. State of the Art.* Verlag Integrative Psychiatrie, Vienna, pp. 53–75.

Hoffmann, K. and Priebe, S. (1996). Welche Bedürfnisse nach Hilfe haben schizophrene Lang-zeitpatienten? – Probleme der Selbst – und Fremdbeurteilung von 'Needs'. *Fortschritte der eurologie Psychiatrie*, 64, 473–481.

Hoffmann, K., Isermann, M., Kaiser, W. and Priebe, S. (1997). Lebensqualität, Bedürfnisse und Behandlungsbewertung langzeithospitalisierter Patienten. Teil II der Berliner Enthospitalisie rungsstudie. *Psychiatrische Praxis*, 24, 221–226.

Hoffmann, K., Kaiser, W., Isermann, M. and Priebe, S. (1998). Wie verändert sich die Lebensqualität langzeithospitalisierter psychiatrischer Patienten nach ihrer Entlassung in die Gemeinde? *Gesundheitswesen*, 60, 232–238.

Hofstätter, P.R. (1986). *Foundations of Satisfaction.* Fromm, Osnabrück.

Hogan, T.P. and Awad, A.G. (1992). Subjective response to neuroleptics and outcome in schizophrenia: a re-examination comparing two measures. *Psychological Medicine*, **22**, 347–452.

Hogan, T.P., Awad, A.G. and Eastwood, M.R. (1983). A self-report scale predictive of drug compliance in schizophrenia: reliability and discriminative ability. *Psychological Medicine*, **13**, 177–183.

Holloway, F. (1991). Day care in an inner city – II, quality of services. *British Journal of Psychiatry*, **158**, 810–816.

Holloway, F. (1994). Need in community psychiatry: a consensus is required. *Psychiatric Bulletin*, **8**, 321–323.

Holloway, F. (1996a). Community psychiatric care: from libertarianism to coercion: 'moral panic' and mental health policy in Britain. *Health Care Analysis*, **4**, 235–243.

Holloway, F. (1996b). The quality of life of long-term psychiatric day patients: an exploratory study of the impact of clinical factors on quality of life. *Social Work and Social Sciences Review*, **6**, 110–116.

Holloway, F. and Carson, J. (1998). Intensive case management for the severely mentally ill: a controlled trial. *British Journal of Psychiatry*, **172**, 19–22.

Holloway, F., Murray, M., Squire, C. and Carson, J. (1996). Intensive case management: putting it into practice. *Psychiatric Bulletin*, **20**, 395–397.

Hornquist, J.O., Wikby, A., Hansson, B. and Andersson, P.O. (1993). Quality of life: status and change (QLSC): reliability, validity and sensitivity of a generic assessment approach tailored for diabetes. *Quality of Life Research*, **2**, 263–279.

Hoult, J. (1986). Community care of the acutely mentally ill. *British Journal of Psychiatry*, **149**, 137–144.

Huxley, P.J. (1993). Systematic assessment methods in psychiatric social work. In: Granville-Grossman, K. (Ed.), *Recent Advances in Clinical Psychiatry*. Churchill Livingstone, Edinburgh/London.

Huxley, P.J. (1998). Are objective and subjective well-being related? Paper presented at the 12th European Health Psychology Conference, Vienna, September 1998.

Huxley, P. and Warner, R. (1992). Case management, quality of life, and satisfaction with services of long-term psychiatric patients. *Hospital and Community Psychiatry*, **43**, 799–802.

Hyland, M.E., Finnis, S. and Irvine, S.H. (1991). A scale for assessing quality of life in adult asthma sufferers. *Journal of Psychosomatic Research*, **35**, 99–110.

Jaeschke, R. and Guyatt, G.H. (1990). How to develop and validate a new quality of life instrument. In: Spilker, B. (Ed.), *Quality of Life Assessments in Clinical Trials*. Raven, New York, pp. 47–57.

Jerrell, J. and Hu, T.W. (1989). Cost-effectiveness of intensive clinical and case management compared with an existing system of care. *Inquiry*, **26**, 224–234.

Jerrell, J. and Ridgley, M.S. (1995). Comparative effectiveness of three approaches to serving people with severe mental illness and substance abuse disorders. *Journal of Nervous and Mental Disease*, **183**, 566–576.

Joyce, C.R.B. (1988). Quality of life: the state of the art in clinical assessment. In: Walker, S.R. and Rosser, R.M. (Eds). *Quality of Life: Assessment and Application*. MTP-Press, Lancaster, pp. 169–179.

Kaiser, W. and Priebe, S. (1998). On the measurement of long-term and short-term change of subjective quality of life in chronic schizophrenic patients. *Der Nervenarzt*, **69**, 219–227.

Kaiser, W., Priebe, S., Hoffmann, K. and Isermann, M. (1996). Subjektive Lebensqualität bei Patienten mit chronischer Schizophrenie. *Der Nervenarzt*, **67**, 6572–582.

Kaiser, W., Priebe, S., Barr, W., Hoffmann, K., Isermann, M., Roder-Wanner, U. and Huxley, P.J. (1997). Profiles of subjective quality of life in schizophrenic in-patient and outpatient samples. *Psychiatry Research*, **66**, 153–166.

Kaiser, W., Burow, S., Dahms, M., Lund, H., Nast, J. and Zindel, K. (1998a). Interviewer-Effekte bei der Erhebung subjektiver Lebensqualität und der Zufriedenheit mit der Betreuung im Betreuten Wohnen. *Psychiatrische Praxis*, **25**, 142–148.

Kaiser, W., Hoffmann, K., Isermann, M. and Priebe, S. (1998b). Behandlerprognosen und Entlassungen nach 2 Jahren. Teil III der Berliner Enthospitalisierungsstudie. *Psychiatrische Praxis*, **25**, 67–71.

Katschnig, H. (1997). How useful is the concept of quality of life in psychiatry? *Current Opinion in Psychiatry*, **10**, 337–345.

Katschnig, H., Freeman, H. and Sartorius, N. (Eds) (1997). *Quality of Life in Mental Disorders*. Wiley, Chichester.

Katz, S. (1987). The science of quality of life. *Journal of Chronic Diseases*, **40**, 459–463.

Kearns, R., Taylor, S.M. and Dear, M. (1987). Coping and satisfaction among the chronically mentally disabled. *Canadian Journal of Community Mental Health*, **6**, 13–24.

Kellner, R. and Sheffield, B.F. (1973). A self rating scale of distress. *Psychological Medicine*, **3**, 88–100.

Kilian, R. (1995). Ist Lebensqualität meßbar? Probleme der quantitativen und Möglichkeiten der qualitativen Erfas-sung von Lebensqualität in der Psychiatrie. *Psychiatrische Praxis*, **22**, 97–101.

King, D.J. (1990). The effect of neuroleptics on cognitive and psychomotor function. *British Journal of Psychiatry*, **157**, 799–811.

Kühn, A., Rosendahl, W. and Henning, H. (1997). Lebensqualität und Alltagsbewältigung chronisch schizophrener Patienten. Ergebnisse einer qualitativen Pilotstudie. *Psychotherapie, Psychosomatik und medizinische Psychologie*, **47**, 64–71.

Lafave, H.G., de Sauza, H.R. and Gerber, G.J. (1996). Assertive community treatment of severe mental illness: a Canadian experience. *Psychiatric Services*, **47**, 757–759.

Lauer, G. (1993). Ergebnisse der Lebensqualitätforschung bei chronisch psychisch Kranken. *Psychiatrische Praxis*, **20**, 88–90.

Lauer, G. (1994a). Chronisch psychisch Kranke: Ergebnisse und Probleme der Lebensqualitätsperspektive. *Deutsches Ärzteblatt*, **91**, 914–915.

Lauer, G. (1994b). The quality of life issue in chronic mental illness. In: Dauwalder, J.P. (Ed.), *Psychology and Promotion of Health*. Swiss Monographs in Psychology. No. 2. Hogrefe and Huber, Seattle, pp. 28–34.

Lauer, G. (1995). Die Lebensqualität psychiatrischer Patienten: Theoretische Grundlagen, empirische Resultate und Implikationen für die weitere Forschung. In: Pawlik, K. (Ed), *Bericht über den 39. Kongreß der Deutschen Gesellschaft für Psychologie in Hamburg 1994*. Hogrefe, Göttingen, pp. 357–362.

Lauer, G. (1996). Lebensqualität und Schizophrenie: Ein Überblick über empirische Ergebnisse. In: Möller, H.-J., Engel, R.R. and Hoff, P. (Eds), *Befunderhebung in der Psychiatrie: Lebensqualität, Negativsymptomatik und andere aktuelle Entwicklungen*. Springer, Vienna, pp. 63–71.

Lauer, G. (1997a). Zur Lebensqualität psychiatrischer Patienten. *Report Psychologie*, **22**, 122–126.

Lauer, G. (1997b) Lebensqualitätsunterschiede unter klassischen versus atypischen Neuroleptika. Paper, presented at: Winterseminar für Biologische Psychiatrie, Oberlech, Austria.

Lauer, G. (1997c). Die Lebensqualitätsperspektive in der Psychiatrie: Ein kritischer Überblick. *Verhaltenstherapie & psychosoziale Praxis*, **29**, 391–405.

Lauer, G. (1997d). Lebensqualität als Outcome-Kriterium. In: Mundt, C., Linden, M. and Barnett, W. (Eds), *Psychotherapie in der Psychiatrie*. Springer, Vienna, pp. 392–395, 451–454.

Lauer, G. (1999a). Die Lebensqualitätsdimension in der Qualitätssicherung. In: Laireiter, A.R. and Vogel, H. (Eds), *Qualitätssicherung in der Psychotherapie – Ein Werkstattbuch*. DGVT-Verlag, Tübingen, in press.

Lauer, G. (1999b). Die Lebensqualität psychiatrischer Patienten: Überblick über eine sich differenzierende Forschungslandschaft. *Fortschritte der Neurologie Psychiatrie*, in preparation.

Lauer, G. and Bähr, G. (1998). Lebensqualität und Neuroleptikanebenwirkungen bei Chronisch Schizophrenen: Eine Querschnittsstudie. *Report Psychologie*, **23**, 642–646.

Lauer, G. and Sellmann, R. (1993). Lebensqualität und Selbstkonzept bei Chronisch Psychisch Kranken. In: Baumgärtel, F. and Wilker, F.W. (Eds), *Klinische Psychologie im Spiegel ihrer Praxis*. Deutscher Psychologen Verlag, Bonn, pp. 95–98.

Lauer, G. and Schneider, G. (1995). Europäische und amerikanische Ergebnisse zur Frage der Lebensqualität chronisch Psychisch Kranker. In: Wetter, U. and Wilker, F.W. (Eds), *Europa – Der Mensch im Mittelpunkt*. Deutscher Psychologen Verlag, Bonn, pp. 91–102.

Lauer, G. and Stegmüller-Koenemund, U. (1994). Bereichsspezifische subjektive Lebensqualität und krankheitsbedingte Einschränkungen chronisch schizophrener Patienten. *Psychiatrische Praxis*, **21**, 70–73.

Leff, J. (Ed.) (1993). Evaluating the transfer of care from psychiatric hospitals to district based services. *British Journal of Psychiatry*, **162**, (Suppl. 19), 6.

Lehman, A.F. (1983a). The well-being of chronic mental patients. Assessing their quality of life. *Archives of General Psychiatry*, **40**, 369–373.

Lehman, A.F. (1983b). The effects of psychiatric symptoms on quality of life assessments among the chronic mentally ill. *Evaluation and Programme Planning*, **6**, 143–151.

Lehman, A.F. (1986). The quality of life of chronic patients in a state hospital and in community residences. *Hospital and Community Psychiatry*, **37**, 901–907.

Lehman, A.F. (1988). A quality of life interview for the chronically mentally ill. *Evaluation and Program Planning*, **11**, 51–62.

Lehman, A.F. (1996). Measures of quality of life among persons with severe and persistent mental disorders. *Social Psychiatry and Psychiatric Epidemiology*, **31**, 78–88.

Lehman, A.F. (1997). Instruments for measuring quality of life in mental illnesses. In: Katschnig, H., Freeman, H. and Sartorius, N. (Eds). *Quality of Life in Mental Disorders*. Wiley, Chichester, pp. 79–94.

Lehman, A.F. and Burns, B.J. (1990). Severe mental illness in the community. In: Spilker, B. (Ed.), *Quality of Life Assessments in Clinical Trials*. Raven, New York, pp. 357–366.

Lehman, A.F., Ward, N.C. and Linn, L.C. (1982). Chronic mental patients: the quality of life issue. *American Journal of Psychiatry*, **139**, 1271–1275.

Lehman, A.F., Possidente, S. and Hawker, F. (1986). The quality of life in a state hospital and in community residences. *Hospital and Community Psychiatry*, **37**, 901–907.

Lehman, A.F., Slaughter, J.G. and Myers, C.P. (1991). Quality of life in alternative residential settings. *Psychiatric Quarterly*, **62**, 35–49.

Lehman, A.F., Slaughter, J.G. and Myers, C.P. (1992). Quality of life experiences of the chronically mentally ill: gender and stages of life effects. *Evaluation and Program Planning*, **15**, 7–12.

Lehman, A.F., Herron, J.D., Schwartz, R.P. and Myers, C.P. (1993). Rehabilitation for adults with severe mental illness and substance use disorders: a clinical trial. *Journal of Nervous and Mental Disease*, **181**, 86–90.

Lehman, A.F., Postrado, L.T., McNary, S.W. and Goldman, H.H. (1994). Continuity of care and client outcomes in the Robert Wood Johnson Foundation programme on chronic mental illness. *Milbank Quarterly*, **72**, 105–122.

Lehman, A.F., Kernan, E., Deforge, B.R. and Dixon, L. (1995a). Effects of homelessness on the quality of life of persons with severe mental illness. *Psychiatric Services*, **46**, 922–926.

Lehman, A.F., Rachuba, L.T. and Postrado, L.T. (1995b). Demographic influences on quality of life among persons with chronic mental illness. *Evaluation and Programme Planning*, **18**, 155–164.

Lehman, A.F., Dixon, L.B., Kernan, E. and Deforge, B. (1997). A randomised trial of assertive community treatment for homeless persons with severe mental illness. *Archives of General Psychiatry*, **54**, 1038–1043.

Leimkühler, A.M. and Müller, U. (1996). Patient satisfaction – artefact or social fact. *Der Nervenarzt*, 67, 765–773.

Lepkifker, E., Horesh, N. and Floru, S. (1988). Life satisfaction and adjustment in lithium-treated affective patients in remission. *Acta Psychiatrica Scandinavica*, 78, 391–395.

Lett, J. (1990). Emics and etics: notes on the epistemology of anthropology. In: Headland, T.N., Pike, K.L. and Harris, M. (Eds), *Emics And Etics: The Insider/Outsider Debate*. Sage, London, pp. 127–142.

Levi, L. and Andersson, L. (1975). *Psychosocial Stress: Population, Environment and Quality of Life*. Spectrum, New York.

Levitt, A.J., Hogan, T.P. and Bucosky, C.M. (1990). Quality of life in chronically mentally ill patients in day treatment. *Psychological Medicine*, 20, 703–710.

Lienert, G.A. (1969). *Construction and Analysis of Tests*. Beltz, Weinheim, Berlin, Basel.

Linn, M.W., Sculthorpe, W.B., Evje, M., Slater, P.H. and Goodman, S.P. (1969). A social dysfunction rating scale. *Journal of Psychiatric Research*, 6, 299–306.

McCarthy, J. and Nelson, G. (1991). An evaluation of supportive housing for current and former psychiatric patients. *Hospital and Community Psychiatry*, 42, 1254–1256.

McGrew, J.H., Bond, G.R., Dietzen, L., McKasson, M. and Miller, L.D. (1995). A multi-site study of client outcomes in assertive community treatment. *Psychiatric Services*, 46, 696–701.

McNair, D.M., Lorr, M. and Droppleman, L.F. (1971). *Manual for the Profile of Mood States*. Educational and Industrial Testing Services, San Diego.

McWalter, G., Toner, H., Corser, A. *et al.* (1994). Needs assessment: their components and definitions with reference to dementia. *Health and Social Care*, 2, 213–219.

Malm, U., May, P.R. and Dencker, S.J. (1981). Evaluation of the quality of life of schizophrenic outpatients: a checklist. *Schizophrenia Bulletin*, 7, 477–487.

Marshall, M., Hogg, L., Lockwood, A. and Gath, D. (1995a). The cardinal needs schedule: a modified version of the MRC needs for care schedule. *Psychological Medicine*, 25, 605–617.

Marshall, M., Lockwood, A. and Gath, D. (1995b). Social services case-management for long term mental disorders: a randomised controlled trial. *The Lancet*, 345, 409–412.

Maslow, A. (1954). *Motivation and Personality*. Harper and Row, New York.

May, P.R.A. (1986). Some research relating to the treatment of Bleuler's disease (schizophrenia). *Psychiatric Journal of the University of Ottawa*, 11, 117–126.

Mayers, C.A. (1995). Defining and assessing quality of life. *British Journal of Occupational Therapy*, 58, 146–150.

Mechanic, D. (1997). Organization of care and quality of life of persons with serious and persistent mental illness. In: Katschnig, H., Freeman, H. and Sartorius, N. (Eds), *Quality of Life in Mental Disorders*. Wiley, Chichester, pp. 305–317.

Mechanic, D., McAlpine, D., Rosenfield, S. and Davis, D. (1994). Effects of illness attribution and depression on the quality of life among persons with serious mental illness. *Social Science and Medicine*, 39, 155–164.

Meltzer, H.Y., Burnett, S., Bastani, B. and Ramirez, L.F. (1990). Effects of six months of clozapine treatment on the quality of life of chronic schizophrenic patients. *Hospital of Community Psychiatry*, 41, 892–897.

Meltzer, H.Y., Cola, P., Way, L., Thompson, P.A., Bastani, B., Davies, M.A. and Snitz, B. (1993). Cost effectiveness of clozapine in neuroleptic-resistant schizophrenia. *American Journal of Psychiatry*, 150, 1630–1638.

Mercier, C. and Filion, J. (1987). La qualité de la vie: perspectives théoretiques et empiriques (English Summary). *Santé mentale au Quebec*, 12, 135–143.

Mercier, C. and King, S. (1994). A latent variable causal model of the quality of life and community tenure of psychotic patients. *Acta Psychiatrica Scandinavica*, 89, 72–77.

Michalos, A.C. (1986). Job satisfaction, marital satisfaction, and the quality of life: A review and a preview. In: Andrews, F.M. (Ed.), *Research on the Quality of Life*. University of Michigan, Institute for Social Research, Ann Arbor, pp. 57–82.

Missenden, K., Oliver, N., Carson, J., Holloway, F., Towey, A., Dunn, L. and Collins, E. (1996). Understanding quality of life: a comparison between staff and patients. *Social Work and Social Sciences Review*, 6, 117–129.

Modcrin, M., Rapp, C.A. and Poertner, J. (1988). The evaluation of case management services with the chronically mentally ill. *Evaluation and Programme Planning*, 11, 307–314.

Moeller, H.J., Engel, R.R. and Hoff, P. (Eds). (1996). *Quality of Life, Negative Symptoms and Other Trends*. Springer, Vienna, New York.

Morrow, G.R., Chiarello, J. and Derogatis, L.R. (1978). A new scale for assessing patients' psychosocial adjustment to medical illness. *Psychological Medicine*, 8, 605–610.

Mueser, K.T., Bond, G.R., Drake, R.E. and Resnick, S.G. (1998). Models of community care for severe mental illness: a review of research on case management. *Schizophrenia Bulletin*, 24, 37–74.

Muldoon, M.F., Barger, S.D., Flory, J.D. and Manuck, S.B. (1998). What are quality of life measurements measuring? *British Medical Journal*, 316, 549–545.

Mulkern, V.M. and Manderschield, R.M.N. (1989). Characteristics of community support programme clients in 1980 and 1984. *Hospital and Community Psychiatry*, 40, 165–172.

Mulkern, V., Agosta, J.M., Ashbaugh, J.W. et al. (1986). *Community Support Programme Client Follow Up Study*. Report to NIMH Rockville, Maryland, USA.

Murray, M., Walker, H.W., Mitchell, C. and Pelosi, A. (1996). Needs for care from a demand led community psychiatric service: a study of patients with major mental illness. *British Medical Journal*, 312, 1582–1586.

Naber, D., Walther, A., Kirshere, T. et al. (1995). Subjective effects of neuroleptics predict compliance. In: Gaebel, W. and Awad, A.G. (Eds), *Prediction of Neuroleptic Treatment Outcome in Schizophrenia: Concepts and Methods*. Springer Verlag, Vienna, pp. 111–122.

Naess, S. (1994). Does self-deception enhance the quality of life? In: Nordenfelt, L. (Ed.), *Concepts and Measurement of Quality of Life in Health Care*. Kluwer, Dordrecht.

Nagpal, R. and Sell, H. (1985). *Subjective Well-being*. SEARO Regional Health Papers No. 7.

Najman, J.M. and Levine, S. (1981). Evaluating the impact of medical care and technologies on the quality of life: a review and critique. *Social Science and Medicine*, 15, 107–115.

National Health Service Executive (1998). *The new NHS, modern and dependable: a national framework for assessing performance*. Consultation document. Department of Health, London.

Niemi, M.L., Laaksonen, R., Kotila, M. and Waltimo, O. (1988). Quality of life 4 years after stroke. *Stroke*, 19, 1101–1107.

Nocon, A. and Quershi, H. (1996). *Outcomes of Community Care for Users and Carers*. Open University Press, Milton Keynes.

Norman, I. and Parker, F. (1990). Psychiatric patients' views of their lives before and after moving to a hostel: a qualitative study. *Journal of Advanced Nursing*, 15, 1036–1044.

Nunally, J.C. (1978). *Psychometric Theory*. 2nd edn. McGraw-Hill, New York.

O'Conner-Griffin, B. (1990). Measures of quality of life in persons with severe psychiatric disability. Masters thesis, Dept of Psychology, Indiana University–Purdue University, Indianapolis.

O'Driscoll, C. (1993). The TAPS project 7: mental hospital closure – a literature review of outcome studies and evaluative techniques. *British Journal of Psychiatry*, 162 (Suppl. 19), 7–17.

Office of Technology Assessment (OTA). (1988). *The Quality of Medical Care: Information for Consumers*. Congress of the United States, Washington.

Okin, R.L. and Pearsall, D. (1993). Patients' perceptions of their quality of life 11 years after discharge from a state hospital. *Hospital and Community Psychiatry*, 44, 236–240.

Okin, R.L., Borus, J.F., Baer, L. and Jones, A.L. (1995). Long-term outcome of state hospital patients discharged into structured community residential settings. *Psychiatric Services*, **46**, 73–78.

Okun, M.A. and Stock, W.A. (1987). The construct validity of subjective well-being measures: an assessment via quantitative research syntheses. *Journal of Community Psychology*, **15**, 481–492.

Okun, M.A., Stock, W.A., Haring, M.J. and Witter, R.A. (1984). Health and subjective well-being: a meta-analysis. *International Journal of Aging and Human Development*, **19**, 111–132.

Oldridge, M.L. and Hughes, I.C.T. (1992). Psychological well-being in families with a member suffering from schizophrenia. An investigation into long-standing problems. *British Journal of Psychiatry*, **161**, 249–251.

Olfson, M. (1990). Assertive community treatment: an evaluation of the experimental evidence. *Hospital and Community Psychiatry*, **41**, 634–641.

Oliver, J.P.J. (1991a). The social care directive: development of a quality of life profile for use in community services for the mentally ill. *Social Work and Social Sciences Review*, **3**, 5–45.

Oliver, J.P.J. (1991b). The quality of life in community care: a consideration of hostel wards prompted by a survey of residential facilities. In: Young, R. (Ed.), *Residential Needs for Severely Disabled Psychiatric Patients: The Case for Hospital Hostels*. HMSO, London, pp. 53–60.

Oliver, J.P.J. and Mohamad, H. (1992). The quality of life of the chronically mentally ill: a comparison of public, private, voluntary residential provisions. *British Journal of Social Work*, **22**, 391–404.

Oliver, J.P.J., Huxley, P.J., Bridges, K. and Mohamad, H. (1996). *Quality of Life and Mental Health Services*. Routledge, London.

Oliver, J.P.J., Huxley, P.J., Priebe, S. and Kaiser, W. (1997). Measuring the quality of life of severely mentally ill people using the Lancashire Quality of Life Profile. *Social Psychiatry and Psychiatric Epidemiology*, **32**, 76–83.

Oliver, N., Holloway, F. and Carson, J. (1995). Deconstructing quality of life. *Journal of Mental Health*, **4**, 1–4.

Orley, J., Saxena, S. and Herrman, H. (1998). Quality of life and mental illness. *British Journal of Psychiatry*, **172**, 291–293.

Overall, J.E. and Gorham, D.R. (1962). The Brief Psychiatric Rating Scale. *Psychological Report*, **10**, 799–812.

Parloff, M.B., Kelman, H.C. and Frank, J.D. (1954). Comfort, effectiveness and self-awareness as criteria of improvement in psychotherapy. *American Journal of Psychiatry*, **111**, 343–351.

Paykel, E.S., Weissman, M., Prusoff, B.A. and Tonks, C.M. (1971). Dimensions of social adjustment in depressed women. *Journal of Nervous and Mental Diseases*, **152**, 158–172.

Peduzzi, P., Hultgren, H., Thomsen, J. and Detre, K. (1987). Ten-year effect of medical and surgical therapy on quality of life: Veterans Administration cooperative study of coronary artery surgery. *The American Journal of Cardiology*, **59**, 1017–1023.

Petch, E. and Bradley, C. (1997). Learning the lessons from homicide inquiries: adding insult to injury? *Journal of Forensic Psychiatry*, **8**, 161–184.

Phelan, M., Slade, M., Thornicroft, G. *et al.* (1995). The Camberwell Assessment of Need: the validity and reliability of an instrument to assess the needs of people with severe mental illness. *British Journal of Psychiatry*, **1676**, 589–595.

Pike, K.L. (1967). *Language in Relation to a Unified Theory of Structure of Human Behavior, 2nd edn.* Mouton, The Hague.

Pike, K.L. (1990). On the emics and etics of Pike and Harris. In: Headland, T.N., Pike, K.L. and Harris, M. (Eds), *Emics and Etics: The Insider/Outsider Debate*. Russell Sage Foundation, London, pp. 28–47.

Pinkney, A.A., Gerber, G.J. and Lafave, H.G. (1991). Quality of life after psychiatric rehabilitation: the clients' perspective. *Acta Psychiatrica Scandinavica*, **83**, 86–91.

Postrado, L.T. and Lehman, A.F. (1995). Quality of life and clinical predictors of rehospitalization of persons with severe mental illness. *Psychiatric Services*, **46**, 1161–1165.

Priebe, S. (1994). Bedeutung der Lebensqualität für psychiatrische Versorgung und Forschung. *Psychiatrische Praxis*, **21**, 87.

Priebe, S., Gruyters, T., Heinze, M., Hoffmann, C. and Jäkel, A. (1995). Subjektive Evaluationskriterien in der psychiatrischen Versorgung – Erhebungsmethoden für Forschung und Praxis. *Psychiatrische Praxis*, **22**, 140–144.

Priebe, S., Hoffmann, K., Isermann, M. and Kaiser, W. (1996). Klinische Merkmale langzeithospitalisierter Patienten – Teil I der Berliner Enthospitalisierungsstudie. *Psychiatrische Praxis*, **23**, 15–20.

Priebe, S., Warner, R., Hubschmid, T. and Eckle, I. (1998a). Employment, attitudes toward work, and quality of life among people with schizophrenia in three countries. *Schizophrenia Bulletin*, **24**, 469–476.

Priebe, S., Kaiser, W., Huxley, P.J., Röder-Wanner, U. and Rudolf, H. (1998b). Do different subjective evaluation criteria reflect distinct constructs? *Journal for Nervous and Mental Disease*, **186**, 385–392.

Priebe, S., Huxley, P., Knight, S. and Evans, S. (1999a). Application and results of the Manchester Short Assessment of Quality of Life (MANSA). *The International Journal of Social Psychiatry*, in press.

Priebe, S., Röder-Wanner, U. and Kaiser, W. (1999b). Quality of life in first admitted schizophrenia patients. *Psychological Medicine*, in press.

Prism Conference. (1997). Evaluation Results Presented At The Prism Conference, London.

Raphael, D. (1996). Defining quality of life: eleven debates concerning its measurement. In: Renwick, R., Brown, I. and Nagler, M. (Eds), *Quality of Life in Health Promotion and Rehabilitation. Conceptual Approaches, Issues, and Applications*. Russell Sage Foundation, Thousand Oaks, pp. 146–165.

Rawlinson, J.W. and Brown, A.C. (1991). Community psychiatric nursing in Britain. In: Bennett, D.H. and Freeman, H.L. (Eds), *Community Psychiatry*. Churchill Livingstone, Edinburgh.

Renwick, R. and Brown, I. (1996). The Centre for Health Promotion's conceptual approach to quality of life: being, belonging, and becoming. In: Renwick, R., Brown, I. and Nagler, M. (Eds), *Quality of Life in Health Promotion and Rehabilitation. Conceptual Approaches, Issues, and Applications*. Russell Sage Foundation, Thousand Oaks, pp. 75–86.

Renwick, R. and Friefeld, S. (1996). Quality of life and rehabilitation. In: Renwick, R., Brown, I. and Nagler, M. (Eds), *Quality of Life in Health Promotion and Rehabilitation. Conceptual Approaches, Issues, and Applications*. Russell Sage Foundation, Thousand Oaks, pp. 26–36.

Research and Education Association (1981). *Handbook of Psychiatric Rating Scales*. Research and Education Association, New York.

Revicki, R.A., Haley, S., Hamilton, L. *et al.* (1997). Quality of life outcomes for olanzepine and haloperidol treatment for schizophrenia and other psychotic disorders: results of an international randomised clinical trial. *Quality of Life Research*, **6**, 708.

Röder-Wanner, U.-U. and Priebe, S. (1998). Objective and subjective quality of life of first-admitted women and men with schizophrenia. *European Archives of Psychiatry and Clinical Neurosciences*, **248**, 250–258.

Rosenberg, M. (1965). *Society And The Adolescent Self-Image*. Princeton University Press, Princeton, NJ.

Rosenheck, R., Tekell, J., Peters, J., Cramer, J., Fontana, A., Zxu, W., Thomas, J., Henderson, W. and Charney, D. (1998). Does participation in psychosocial treatment augment the benefit of clozapine? *Archives of General Psychiatry*, **55**, 618–625.

Rosser, R.M., Cottee, M., Rabin, R. and Selai, C. (1992). Index of health related quality of life. In: Hopkins, A. (Ed.), *Measures of the Quality of Life and the Uses to which Such Measures May Be Put*. Royal College of Physicians, London.

Rossi, P.H., Freeman, H.E. and Hoffmann, G. (1988). *Programme Evaluation: Einführung in die Methoden angewandter Sozialforschung*. Enke, Stuttgart.

Royal Pharmaceutical Society of Great Britain (1997). *From Compliance to Concordance: Achieving Shared Goals in Medicine Taking*. RPSGB and Merck, Sharp & Dohme, London.

Rudolf, H. and Priebe, S. (1999). Subjektive Lebensqualität und Stellenwert Unterschiedlicher Lebensbereiche bei Alkoholabhängigen Frauen. *Psychiatrische Praxis*, in press.

Rudolf, H., Bommer, I. and Priebe, S. (1996). Alkoholabhängige Frauen nach der körperlichen Entgiftung – Wie bewerten sie ihre Lebenssituation? *Wiener Zeitschrift für Suchtforschung*, **19**, 47–53.

Ruggeri, M. (1994). Patients' and relatives' satisfaction with psychiatric services: the state of art of its measurement. *Social Psychiatry and Psychiatric Epidemiology*, **29**, 212–227.

Salvador-Carulla, L. (1997). Measuring quality of life in cost analysis: controversies and use in mental health. In: Katschnig, H., Freeman, H. and Sartorius, N. (Eds), *Quality of Life in Mental Disorders*. Wiley, Chichester, pp. 287–304.

Sanifort, F., Becker, M. and Diamond, R. (1996). Judgements of quality of life of individuals with severe mental disorders: patient self-report versus provider perspectives. *American Journal of Psychiatry*, **153**, 497–502.

Sartorius, N. (1992). Rehabilitation and quality of life. *Hospital and Community Psychiatry*, **43**, 1180–1181.

Schalock, R.L., Keith, K.D., Hoffman, K. and Karan, O.C. (1989). Quality of life: its measurement and use. *Mental Retardation*, **27**, 25–31.

Schipper, H. (1983). Why measure quality of life? *Canadian Medical Association Journal*, **128**, 1367–1370.

Schipper, H., Clinch, J. and Powell, V. (1990). Definitions and conceptual issues. In: Spilker, B. (Ed.), *Quality of Life Assessments in Clinical Trials*. Raven, New York, pp. 11–24.

Schneider, H.J. (1993). Therapieziele und Lebensqualität – philosophische Aspekte. *Fundamenta Psychiatrica*, **7**, 202–207.

Schneider, J. (1993). Care programming in mental health: assimilation and adaptation. *British Journal of Social Work*, **23**, 383–403.

Schulberg, H.C. and Bromet, E. (1981). Strategies for evaluating the outcome of community services for the chronically mentally ill. *American Journal of Psychiatry*, **138**, 930–935.

Schwarz, N., Wänke, M. and Bless, H. (1994). Subjective assessments and evaluations of change: some lessons from social cognition research. In: Stroebe, W. and Hewstone, M. (Eds), *European Review of Social Psychology*. Wiley, New York, pp. 181–210.

Secretaries of State for Health and Social Security, Wales and Scotland. (1989). *Caring for People. Community Care in the Next Decade and Beyond*. HMSO, London.

Segal, S. and Aviram, U. (1977). *Community Based Sheltered Care: A Study of Community Care and Social Integration*. Wiley Interscience, New York.

Shadish, W.R., Orwin, R.G., Silber, B.G. and Bootzin, R.R. (1985). The subjective well-being of mental patients in nursing homes. *Evaluation and Programme Planning*, **8**, 239–250.

Shepherd, G., Muijen, M., Dean, R. and Cooney, R. (1996). Residential care in hospital and in the community – quality of care and quality of life. *British Journal of Psychiatry*, **168**, 448–456.

Simmons, S. (1994). Quality of life in community mental health care – a review. *International Journal of Nursing Studies*, **31**, 183–193.

Simon, M.D. (1997). The quality of life of the relatives of the mentally ill. In: Katschnig, H., Freeman, H. and Sartorius, N. (Eds), *Quality of Life in Mental Disorders*. Wiley, Chichester, pp. 253–260.

Simpson, C.J., Hyde, C.E. and Faragher, E.B. (1989). The chronically mentally ill in community facilities: a study of quality of life. *British Journal of Psychiatry*, **154**, 77–82.

Skantze, K. and Malm, U. (1994). A new approach to facilitation of working alliances based on patients' quality of life goals. *Nordic Journal of Psychiatry*, **48**, 37–55.

Skantze, K., Malm, U., Dencker, S.J. and May, P.R.A. (1990). Quality of life in schizophrenia. *Nordisk Psykiatrisk Tidesskrift*, **44**, 71–75.

Skantze, K., Malm, U., Dencker, S.J., May, P.R. and Corrigan, P. (1992). Comparison of quality of life with standard of living in schizophrenic outpatients. *British Journal of Psychiatry*, **161**, 797–801.

Slevin, M.L., Plant, H., Lynch, D., Drinkwater, J. and Gregory, W.M. (1988). Who should measure quality of life, the doctor or the patient? *British Journal of Cancer*, **57**, 109–112.

Soloman, P. and Draine, J. (1995a). One year outcomes of a randomised trial of case management with seriously mentally ill clients leaving jail. *Evaluation Review*, **19**, 256–273.

Soloman, P. and Draine, J. (1995b). The efficacy of a community case management team: 2-year outcomes of a randomised trial. *Journal of Mental Health Administration*, **22**, 135–146.

Spilker, B. (1990). Introduction. In: Spilker, B. (Ed.), *Quality of Life Assessments in Clinical Trials*. Raven, New York, pp. 3–9.

Spitzer, W.O., Dobson, A.J., Hall, J. *et al.* (1981). Measuring the quality of life of cancer patients. A concise QL-index for use by physicians. *Journal of Chronic Diseases*, **34**, 585–597.

Stein, L.I. and Test, M.A. (1980). Alternative to mental hospital treatment. I, conceptual model, treatment programme and clinical evaluation. *Archives of General Psychiatry*, **37**, 392–397.

Strack, F., Argyle, M. and Schwarz, N. (Eds) (1991). *Subjective Well-Being. An Interdisciplinary Perspective*. Pergamon Press, Oxford.

Strauss, J.S., Rakfeldt, J., Harding, C.M. and Lieberman, P. (1989). Psychological and social aspects of negative symptoms. *British Journal of Psychiatry*, **155**, 128–132.

Sullivan, G. and Lukoff, D. (1990). Sexual side effects of antipsychotic medication: evaluation and interventions. *Hospital and Community Psychiatry*, **41**, 1238–1241.

Sullivan, G., Wells, K.B. and Leake, B. (1991). Quality of life of seriously mentally ill persons in Mississippi. *Hospital and Community Psychiatry*, **42**, 752–755.

Sullivan, G., Wells, K.B. and Leake, B. (1992). Clinical factors associated with better quality of life in a seriously mentally ill population. *Hospital and Community Psychiatry*, **43**, 794–798.

Surles, R.C., Blanch, A.K., Shern, D.L. and Donahue, S.A. (1992). Case management as a strategy for systems change. *Health Affairs*, **11**, 151–163.

Taube, C.A., Morlock, L., Burns, B.J. and Santos, A.B. (1990). New directions in research on assertive community treatment. *Hospital and Community Psychiatry*, **41**, 642–647.

Taylor, R.E., Leese, M., Clarkson, P., Holloway, F. and Thornicroft, G. (1998). Quality of life outcomes for intensive versus standard community mental health services. Prism Psychosis Study. *British Journal of Psychiatry*, **173**, 416–422.

Testa, M.A., Anderson, R.B., Nackley, J.F. and Hollen-Berg, N.K. (1993). The quality of life hypertension study group quality of life and anti-hypertensive therapy in men: a comparison of captopril with enalapril. *New England Journal of Medicine*, **328**, 907–913.

Thornicroft, G. and Breakey, W.R. (1991). The Costar Programme. Improving social network of the long-term mentally ill with a mobile case management service. *British Journal of Psychiatry*, **159**, 245–249.

Torrance, G.W. (1996). Designing and conducting cost-utility analyses. In: Spilker, B. (Ed.), *Quality of Life and Pharmacoeconomics in Clinical Trials*. Lippincott-Raven, Philadelphia.

Van Dam, F.S.A.M., Somers, R. and Van Beek-Couzijn, A.L. (1981). Quality of life: some theoretical issues. *Journal of Clinical Pharmacology* 21, 166–168.

Vandiver, V.L., Diaz, P., Ducunge, E.O. and Castenenda, C. (1993). Cross-cultural quality of life measures with schizophrenic populations: preliminary outcome data from Cuba, Canada, Mexico and USA. Paper, Presented at: 6th Congress of the International Federation of Psychiatric Epidemiology, Lisbon, Portugal, April 14–17 1993.

Van Nieuwenhuizen, C. (1998). *Quality of Life of Persons with Severe Mental Illness: An instrument*. Doctor of Philosophy Thesis, University of Amsterdam, Netherlands.

Van Putten, T. and May, P.R.A. (1978). Subjective response as a predictor of outcome in pharmacotherapy. *Archives of General Psychiatry*, 35, 477–480.

Van Putten, T., May, P.R.A. and Marder, S.R. (1980). Subjective response to thiothixene and chlorpromazine. *Psychopharmacology Bulletin*, 16, 36–38.

Ventura, J., Green, M.F., Shaner, A. and Liberman, R.P. (1993). Training and quality assurance with the Brief Psychiatric Rating Scale: 'the drift busters'. *International Journal of Methods in Psychiatric Research*, 3, 221–244.

Vickrey, B.G., Hays, R.D., Graber, J., Rausch, R., Engel, J.Jr. and Brook, R.H. (1992). A health related quality of life instrument for patients evaluated for epilepsy surgery. *Medical Care*, 30, 99–319.

Vinestock, M. (1996). Risk assessment. 'A word to the wise'? *Advances in Psychiatric Practice*, 2, 3–10.

Voruganti, L.N.P., Malla, A., Cortese, L. and Awad, A.G. (1997). Comparative evaluation of conventional and new anti-psychotic medications with reference to subjective tolerability and side-effects. Proceedings of the 36th Annual Meeting of the American College of Neuropsychopharmacology, 185.

Voruganti, L.N.P., Heslegrave, R.J., Awad, A.G. and Seeman, M. (1998). Quality of life measurement in schizophrenia: reconciling the quest for subjectivity with questions of reliability. *Psychological Medicine*, 28, 165–172.

Waite, A., Carson, J., Cullen, D., Oliver, N. and Holloway, F. (1997). Case management: a week in the life of a clinical case management team. *Journal of Psychiatric and Mental Health Nursing*, 4, 287–294.

Ware, J.E. (1984). Conceptualizing disease impact and treatment outcomes. *Cancer*, 53, 2316–2323.

Warner, R. (1999). The emics and etics of quality of life assessment. *Social Psychiatry and Psychiatric Epidemiology*, in press.

Warner, R. and De Girolamo, G. (1995). *Schizophrenia*. World Health Organization, Geneva.

Warner, R. and Huxley, P.J. (1993). Psychopathology and quality of life among mentally ill patients in the community: British and US samples compared. *British Journal of Psychiatry*, 163, 505–509.

Warner, R., De Girolamo, G. and Belelli, G. (1999). The quality of life of people with schizophrenia in Boulder, Colorado, and Bologna, Italy. *Schizophrenia Bulletin*, in press.

Warr, P. (1978). A study of psychological well-being. *British Journal of Psychology*, 69, 111–121.

Weiss, R. (1974). The provisions of social relationships. In: Rubin, Z. (Ed.), *Doing unto Others*. Prentice Hall, New York.

Wilkinson, G., Williams, B., Krekorian, H., McLees, S. and Falloon, I. (1992). QALYs in Mental Health: a case study. *Psychological Medicine*, 22, 725–731.

Williams, J.I. (1991). Strategies for quality-of-life assessment – a methodologist's view. *Theoretical Surgery*, 6, 152–157.

Williams, R., Walsh, D. and Dalby, J.T. (1992). Services to schizophrenic patients: epidemiological and cost-effectiveness issues. *Irish Journal of Psychological Medicine*, 9, 83–89.

Wing, J.K., Curtis, R.H. and Beevor, A.S. (1996). *Health of the Nation Outcome Scales. Glossary for HoNOS Score Sheet*. The Royal College of Psychiatrists, London.

Wittmann, W.W. (1985). *Evaluationsforschung*. Springer, Berlin, New York, Heidelberg.

Wood, S. and Williams, J.I. (1987). Reintegration to normal living as a proxy to quality of life. *Journal of Chronic Diseases*, **40**, 491–499.

World Health Organization (1948). *Charter*. World Health Organization, Geneva.

World Health Organization (1994). *Quality of Life Assessment. An Annotated Bibliography*. World Health Organization, Geneva.

WHOQOL Group. (1993). *Measuring Quality of Life: The Development of the World Health Organization Quality of Life Instrument (WHOQOL)*. World Health Organization, Geneva.

WHOQOL Group. (1995). The World Health Organization quality of life assessment 6(WHOQOL): position paper. *Social Science and Medicine*, **41**, 1403–1409.

Wright, J.G. and Feinstein, A.R. (1992). A comparative contrast of clinimetric and psychometric methods for constructing indexes and rating scales. *Journal of Clinical Epidemiology*, **45**, 1201–1218.

Wykes, T. (1994). Predicting symptomatic and behavioural outcomes of community care. *British Journal of Psychiatry*, **165**, 486–492.

Zautra, A. and Goodhart, D. (1979). Quality of life indicators: a review of the literature. *Community Mental Health Review*, **4**, 1–10.

Ziebland, S. (1994). Measuring changes in health status. In: Jenkinson, C. (Ed.), *Measuring Health and Medical Outcomes*. VCL Press, London, pp. 42–43.

Zissi, A., Barry, M .M. and Cochrane, R. (1998). A mediational model of quality of life for individuals with severe mental health problems. *Psychological Medicine*, **28**, 1221–1230.

Index

Index